CARDIOVASCULAR

Bayer

BAYER

New Trends in Diagnosis and Management of Stroke

Edited by

K. Poeck E. B. Ringelstein W. Hacke

With Contributions by

G. W. Bielenberg H. K. Breddin G. J. Del Zoppo
H. J. Gelmers K. Gorter W. Hacke L. A. Harker
H. Henningsen C. Kessler G. Korbmacher
J. Krieglstein H. J. Krzywanek J. Marshall
E. B. Ringelstein H.-J. Stierstorfer C. J. de Weerdt
J. H. A. Wiezer H. Zeumer

Springer-Verlag
Berlin Heidelberg New York
London Paris Tokyo

Professor Dr. KLAUS POECK
Professor Dr. ERICH BERND RINGELSTEIN

Abteilung Neurologie der Medizinischen Fakultät
Rheinisch-Westfälische-Hochschule
Pauwelsstraße, D-5100 Aachen

Professor Dr. WERNER HACKE

Abteilung Neurologie, Universität Heidelberg
Kopfklinikum
Im Neuenheimer Feld 400, D-6900 Heidelberg

With 42 Figures

ISBN 3-540-18369-8 Springer-Verlag Berlin Heidelberg New York
ISBN 0-387-18369-8 Springer-Verlag New York Berlin Heidelberg

Library of Congress Cataloging-in-Publication Data. New trends in diagnosis and management of stroke / edited by K. Poeck, E.B. Ringelstein, and W. Hacke; with contributions by G.W. Bielenberg ... [et al.]. p. cm. Bibliography: p. Includes index. ISBN 0-387-18369-8 (U.S.)
1. Cerebrovascular disease – Congresses. I. Poeck, Klaus. II. Ringelstein, E.B. (Erich Bernd), 1948– . III. Hacke, W. (Werner). 1948– .
RC388.5.N475 1987 616.8'1–dc19 87-28454 CIP.

Typesetting: K+V Fotosatz GmbH, D-6124 Beerfelden
Offsetprinting and bookbinding: Druckhaus Beltz, D-6944 Hemsbach/Bergstr.
2125/3130-543210

Preface

It might appear bold to publish the proceedings of yet another symposium on the diagnosis and management of stroke. However, I hope in selecting topics to reflect 'new trends' and in inviting speakers to discuss these trends and the related concepts and results, that we have been successful in attaining a high level of scholarship as well as in appealing to a wide readership.

The central issues here derive from a new typology of strokes that should replace the obsolete distinction based on purely temporal parameters so aptly criticized by Caplan. A classification of strokes on the basis of pathogenesis requires a synopsis of information gained from history, neurological and cardiovascular findings, ultrasound studies (extracranial as well as transcranial), correctly timed CT scan investigation and, if necessary, from selective angiography. Only the recognition of the role of pathogenetic events for a patient permits the application of a rational therapy regimen.

The spectrum of therapy programs ranges from hypervolemic or isovolemic hemodilution, which is indicated by hematological data, to early anticoagulation that has been demonstrated to be safe even in the presence of an ischemic brain lesion. Local intra-arterial fibrinolysis of acute arterial occlusion has proved most beneficial in hindbrain circulation and is applicable also in selected cases of acute occlusion of the proximal segments of the middle cerebral artery. Monitoring of electrophysiological parameters and of arterial perfusion by means of ultrasound techniques is mandatory in these instances. The exact place of calcium entry blockers has yet to be determined. These appear to be very promising agents not only in the early phase after SAH but possibly also in acute ischemic stroke.

A view into the future is provided by contributions on new relatively clot-specific substances with tissue plasminogen activating properties. The many problems involved in this therapeutic approach are probably not yet generally recognized. Selection of patients with angiographically demonstrated acute occlusion of one or more major vessels that explains the patients' signs and symptoms must be achieved; establishment of the proper dosage will be very critical.

Surgical treatment and percutaneous intraluminal angioplasty have not been covered in this symposium, for the emphasis here is on acute stroke, for which these approaches, in spite of their general merit, are rarely if ever employed.

Aachen, October 1987 KLAUS POECK

Acknowledgement

The organizers of the International Symposium on Trends in Diagnosis and Management of Stroke wish to express their gratitude to Bayer AG, Germany, for their generous support which made the organization of the symposium and publication of the proceedings possible.

Contents

Contributors

G. W. Bielenberg, Institute of Pharmacology and Toxicology, FB 16, Philipps-University, Ketzerbach 63, D-3550 Marburg, FRG

H. K. Breddin, Department of Internal Medicine, Division of Angiology, J. W. Goethe-University Hospital, Theodor Stern Kai 7, D-6000 Frankfurt/Main 70, FRG

G. J. Del Zoppo, Department of Basic and Clinical Research, Scripps Clinic and Research Foundation, 10666 North Torrey Pines Road, La Jolla, CA 92037, USA

H. J. Gelmers, Department of Neurology, Streekziekenhuis Almelo, NL-Almelo, The Netherlands

K. Gorter, Department of Neurology, St. Anatonius Ziekenhuis, NL-Sneek, The Netherlands

W. Hacke, Department of Neurology, University of Heidelberg, Kopfklinikum, Im Neuenheimer Feld 400, D-6900 Heidelberg, FRG

L. A. Harker, Department of Basic and Clinical Research, Scripps Clinic and Research Foundation, 10666 North Torrey Pines Road, La Jolla, CA 92037, USA

H. Henningsen, Department of Neurology, University Hospital, Voss-Straße 2, D-6900 Heidelberg 1, FRG

C. Kessler, Department of Neurology, Krankenhaus Merheim, Ostmerheimerstr. 200, D-5000 Köln 91, FRG

Gabriele Korbmacher, Department of Neurology, Klinikum RWTH, University Hospital, D-5100 Aachen, FRG

J. Krieglstein, Institute of Pharmacology and Toxicology, FB 16, Philipps-University, Ketzerbach 63, D-3550 Marburg, FRG

H. J. Krzywanek, Department of Internal Medicine, Division of Angiology, J. W. Goethe-University Hospital, Theodor Stern Kai 7, D-6000 Frankfurt/Main 70, FRG

J. Marshall, Institute of Neurology, National Hospital for Nervous Diseases, Queen Square, London WC1N 3BG, UK

E. B. RINGELSTEIN, Department of Neurology, Klinikum RWTH, University Hospital, D-5100 Aachen, FRG

H.-J. STIERSTORFER, Institute of Pharmacology and Toxicology, FB 16, Philipps-University, Ketzerbach 63, D-3550 Marburg, FRG

C. J. DE WEERDT, Scheper Ziekenhuis, NL-Emmen, The Netherlands

J. H. A. WIEZER, St. Elisabeth Ziekenhuis, NL-Venray, The Netherlands

H. ZEUMER, Department of Neurology, University-Hospital Eppendorf, University of Hamburg, D-2000 Hamburg

Part I
Diagnosis and Pathogenesis of Stroke

Transcranial Doppler Sonography

E. B. RINGELSTEIN [1]

Introduction

Noninvasive techniques nowadays allow a differentiated analysis of stroke patients with respect both to the pathomorphology of ischemic brain lesions and to the underlying arterial disease. The methods employed in this bimodal approach are (a) computerized tomography and, more recently, MRI macroscopic in vivo evaluation of parenchymal brain damage, and (b) Doppler and B-mode ultrasound techniques for identifing causative stenoses and occlusions of brain-supplying arteries and/or cardiac sources of emboli.

Figure 1 indicates that a differentiated view of stroke patients must take account of four different levels of disease manifestation. Intracranial small arteries may be affected by an occlusive process which leads to lacunar infarctions and/or subcortical arteriosclerotic encephalopathy (level 1 in Fig. 1). Due to the small diameter of the penetrating arteries involved, this type of occlusive process cannot be evaluated in vivo by means of cerebral angiography or other angiologic examination techniques but may be visualized only on CT images by means of resulting tissue damage. Until recently, the intracranial occlusive macroangiopathy of the basal cerebral arteries has been a diagnostic gap in ultrasound evaluation (level 2 in Fig. 1). Meanwhile, however, the advent of transcranial Doppler sonography enables one to identify stenosing lesions of these arteries with the help of pulsed Doppler ultrasound. A blind spot nevertheless remains; this lies in the distal branches of the brain-supplying arteries. This problem, however, is clinically of only minor relevance. Occluding lesions of the extracranial brain-supplying arteries can reliably be identified with the help of conventional continuous-wave Doppler sonography or similar diagnostic techniques (level 3 in Fig. 1). In combination with B-mode imaging, any degree of arteriosclerotic lesion can be identified, ranging from nonstenosing plaques and fresh thromboses to pseudo-occlusions and complete occlusions of the neck arteries. Thrombotic processes within the heart can also be diagnosed noninvasively (level 4 in Fig. 1). The majority of large thrombi can be detected with the help of echocardiography including more sophisticated techniques, such as esophageal ultrasound imaging of cardiac valves and contrast echocardiography for the detection of functional right/left shunts via the foramen ovale. Additionally, ^{111}In-labelled platelet scintigraphy also contributes to the identification of thromboembolic disorders of the myocardium and the valvular apparatus (see Kessler and Henningsen, this volume).

---

[1] Department of Neurology, Klinikum RWTH, University Hospital, D-5100 Aachen, FRG

Type of disease		Noninvasive diagnosis with the help of:
Cerebral microangiopathy – Lacunes – Subcortical arteriosclerotic encephalopathy – Basilar brachial occlusion	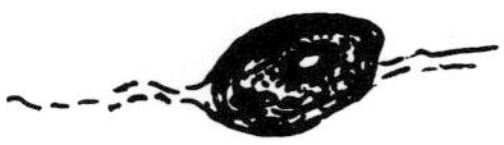	Cranial computerized tomography (CCT) Magnetic resonance imaging (MRI)
Occlusive macroangiopathy of basal cerebral arteries	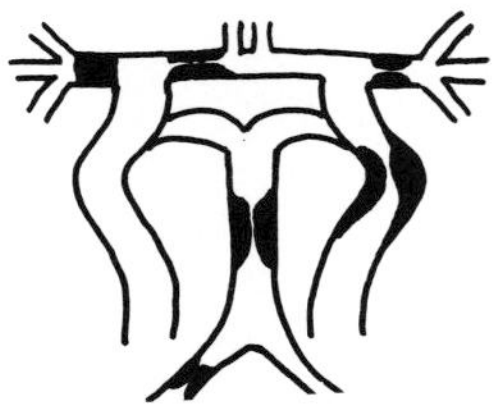	Transcranial Doppler sonography (TCD) including flow mapping of circle of Willis
Occlusive macroangiopathy of extracranial brain-supplying arteries	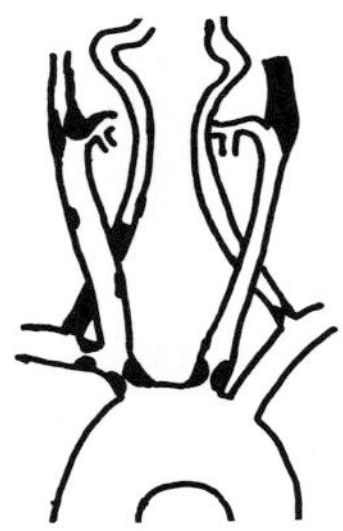	Continuous-wave Doppler ultrasound B-mode impaging (including duplex-scan) Multigate systems Quantitative flow measurement (QFM) Colour-coded flow imaging
Embolizing heart disease	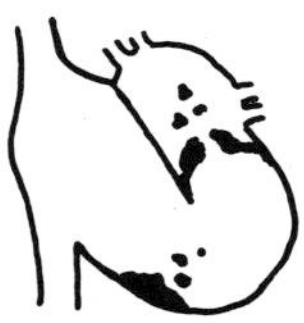	Two-dimensional echocardiography ^{111}In platelet scintigraphy

Fig. 1. Sites of cerebrovascular and cardiac diseases which may cause ischemic stroke

The present article discusses particularly the diagnostic implications of transcranial Doppler sonography (TCD) with respect to occlusive disease of the large basal cerebral arteries (level 2 in Fig. 1) in stroke and stroke-prone patients.

TCD Examination Technique

Principles

TCD was introduced by Rune Aaslid in 1982 as a new noninvasive pulsed Doppler technique [1]. Its principle is demonstrated in Figs. 2, 3. From a transtemporal (Fig. 2), suboccipital (Fig. 3c), transorbital (Fig. 3b) and submandibular approach (Fig. 3a), the basal cerebral arteries can be insonated and tracked into deeper layers with the help of an electronically controlled stepwise movement of the echo-reflecting region of interest (sample volume) within the focus of the beam. This manipulation is called range-gating. The sample volume represents the most sensitive area of the beam; it has a rugbyball-like shape with a lateral diameter of approximately 5 mm and a longitudinal diameter of 10 mm. This sample volume can be moved forward or backward along the various pathways of the intracranial vasculature.

An example of this is the M1 segment of the middle cerebral artery during its insonation at a depth of 50 mm from a transtemporal approach. The corresponding echo is demonstrated in Fig. 2b. At a greater depth, one of approximately 60 mm, the intracranial internal carotid artery (ICA) bifurcation is insonated and a bidirectional flow signal can be received. The upward-deflected curve still represents the signal of the M1 segment of the middle cerebral artery (Fig. 2c) or the sometimes overlapping echo of the C1 segment of the carotid siphon (Fig. 2d), whereas the downward-deflected curve represents the flow signal of the A1 segment of the anterior cerebral artery (Fig. 2c–f). Similar findings can be documented from every part of the circle of Willis and its main branches.

During TCD the transtemporal application is the most informative one. The method and site of probe placement for insonation of the various arterial segments of the intracranial arteries are demonstrated in Fig. 4.

Identification of Skull Window

Several *anatomical obstacles* must be overcome during the application of this new and sophisticated ultrasound technique. The first of these is the identification of a sufficient "ultrasound window" in the temporal region. The transtemporal insonation of the middle cerebral artery should be the first step in the entire procedure; however, the examiner is confronted with the fact that the "ultrasound window" of the temporal bone is extremely variable from individual to individual with respect to size and site, and it may also vary intraindividually from one side of the head to the other. Illustrative temporal ultrasound windows are shown in Fig. 5. As a rule, the probe should be placed immediately frontal to the tragus of the ear and the beam should be directed slightly anteriorly and cephalad with an insonation depth of 50 mm. This is the most promising way in which to receive an MCA signal transtemporally. Once this artery is identified, the circle of Willis – including the top of the basilar artery, the anterior cerebral arteries, the M2 segments of the middle cerebral artery, the C1 segment of the carotid siphon and the P1 and P2 segments of the posterior cerebral artery – can be identified by adjusting the angle of the beam, as well as by stepwise tracking of the basal vascular tree [2, 3].

Identification of Vessel Segments

The next major technical difficulty is the unambiguous identification of distinct vascular segments. Several auxiliary tests may be used to inform the examiner about the exact anatomical position of the sample volume. The *particular vessel segment can be identified* by means of (a) the placement of the probe in the tem-

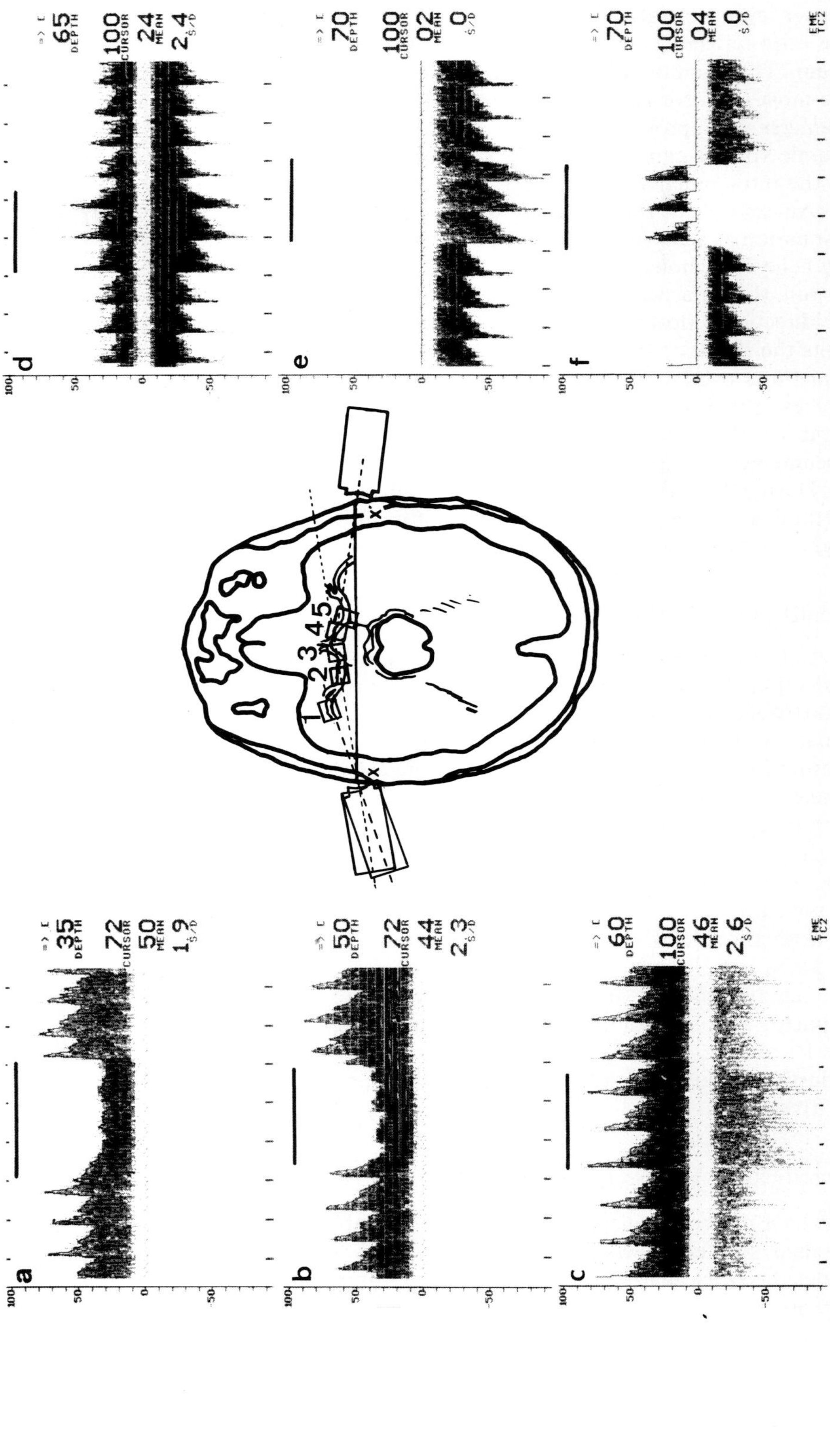
a
35
DEPTH
72
CURSOR
50
MEAN
1.9
S/D
b
50
DEPTH
72
CURSOR
44
MEAN
2.3
S/D
c
60
DEPTH
100
CURSOR
46
MEAN
2.6
S/D
EME
TC2
d
65
DEPTH
100
CURSOR
24
MEAN
2.4
S/D
e
70
DEPTH
100
CURSOR
02
MEAN
0
S/D
f
70
DEPTH
100
CURSOR
04
MEAN
0
S/D
EME
TC2
1
2
3
4
5
x
x

poral, suboccipital, orbital or submandibular position, (b) the direction of the ultrasound beam, (c) the insonation depths, (d) the direction of blood flow, (e) stability of flow signals during forward or backward tracking of the vessel under study, and (f) the effect of compression maneuvers at both neck and facial arteries [2, 3]. The most informative procedure is the use of compression tests on the common carotid artery on either side. However, due to potential risks, these should only be performed where necessary. Table 1 provides the various criteria for identification of the arterial segment under study.

Normal Findings

Neuroradiological material, such as anterior-posterior and lateral-view angiograms, sagittal MRI images, and contrast-medium-enhanced axial CT scans are helpful for the definition of characteristic anatomical landmarks and adequate insonation depths corresponding to the different vessel segments. Some illustrative findings of the carotid system are shown in Fig. 6. Measurements of the vertebrobasilar circulation and its landmarks in 106 MRI scans of normal subjects revealed that the soft tissue in the suboccipital neck region was 30–65 mm thick (mean 50±8 mm), the depth of the vertebrobasilar junction ranged from 70 to 110 mm (mean 84±8 mm) and the top of the basilar artery was found at insonation depths of 90–130 mm (mean 108±8 mm [2]).

Another part of the establishment of practical TCD guidelines has been to define normal flow velocity values within the different vessel segments. This was made during a study on 76 normal subjects of different ages and sex. Representative data are indicated in Fig. 7. Further details are published elsewhere [2, 3, 4].

Fig. 2a–f. Transtemporal insonation of the anterior cerebral circulation. The schematic drawing in the *middle* was reconstructed from an original axial CT scan. *Points X* and *X'* indicate the position of the probe over both temporal "ultrasound windows." During insonation of the anterior (ACA) and middle cerebral arteries (MCA), as well as the C1 segment of the internal carotid artery, the beams are angled slightly frontally. *Numerals 1–5* indicate the sample volumes at different insonations depths.
a At an insonation depth of 35 mm (corresponding to position *1* in the drawing), the M2 segment of the MCA is insonated. *Bar* indicates compression of the ipsilateral common carotid artery, which leads to a dramatic flow velocity reduction. **b** At an insonation depth of 50 mm (corresponding to position *2* in the drawing) the M1 segment of the MCA is insonated. *Bar* indicates compression of the ipsilateral common carotid artery. **c** At an insonation depth of 60 mm (corresponding to position *5* in the drawing) both the MCA and ACA are insonated. *Bar* indicates compression of the contralateral common carotid artery. This compression does not affect blood flow in the MCA, whereas flow velocity in the ACA increases strongly. **d** At an insonation of 65 mm (approximately corresponding to position *4* in the drawing) both the C1 segment of the internal carotid artery (ICA) and the A1 segment of the ACA are insonated. *Bar* indicates compression of the contralateral common carotid artery. In contrast to **c** both arteries reveal a striking increase of flow velocity due to an recruitment of collateral blood flow. **e** At an insonation depth of 70mm (approximately corresponding to position *3* in the drawing) the ACA (A1 segment) is insonated. *Bar* indicates compression of the contralateral common carotid artery which leads to a prompt increase in flow velocity in order to supply the contralateral hemisphere. **f** By contrast, compression of the ipsilateral common carotid artery leads to reversal of blood flow within the A1 segment indicating anterior cross-filling from the contralateral to the ipsilateral hemisphere

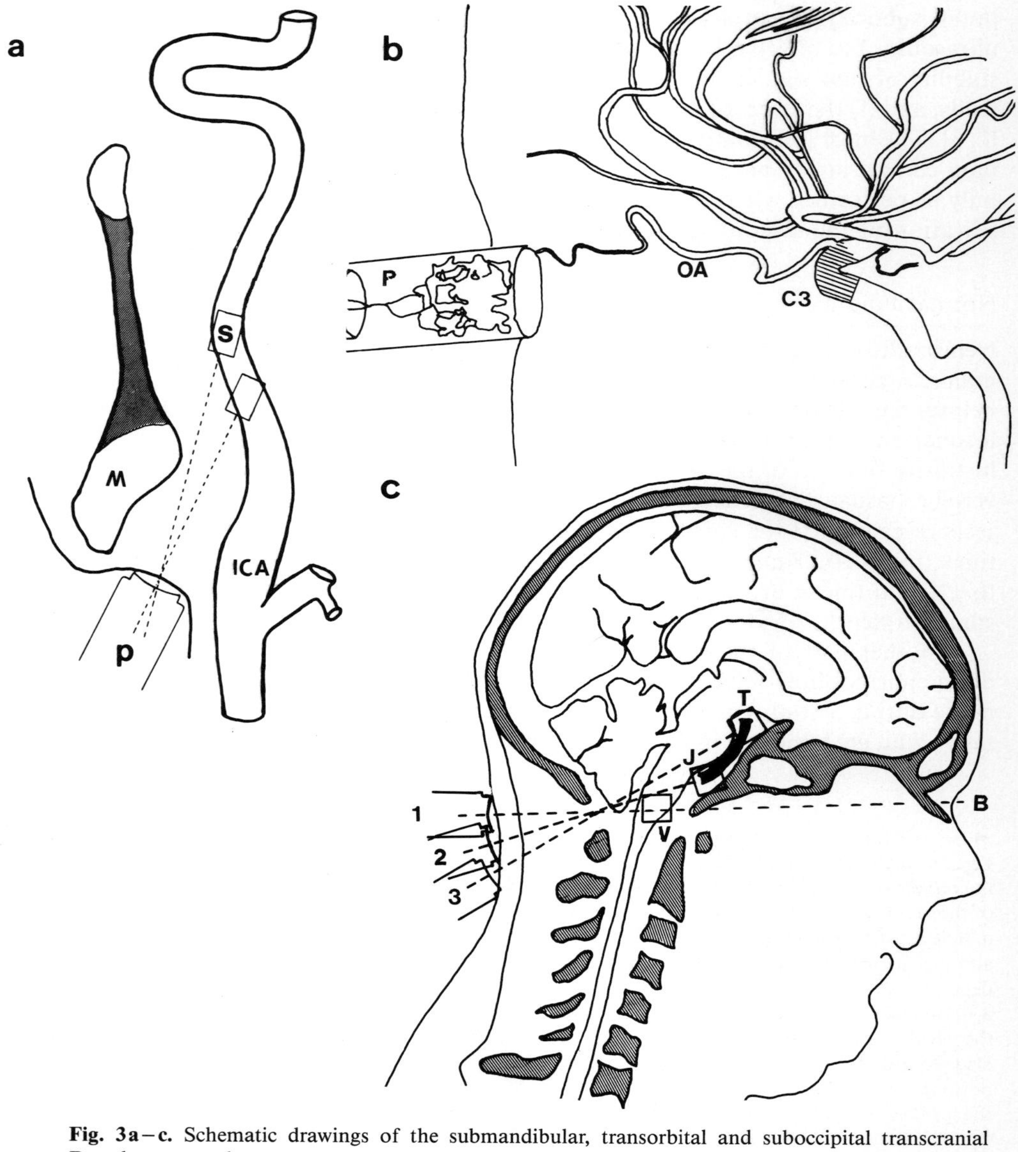

Fig. 3a–c. Schematic drawings of the submandibular, transorbital and suboccipital transcranial Doppler approach.
a From a submandibular position of the probe the retromandibular and intracranial part of the internal carotid artery can be tracked to the petrosal part of the vessel. *P*, probe; *S*, sample volume; *M*, mandible; *ICA* internal carotid artery. **b** Transorbital insonation of the ophthalmic artery (*OA*) and the carotid siphon. *Hatched zone* corresponds to the C3 segment of the internal carotid artery. *P*, probe. The drawing was made from an original angiogram during simultaneous transorbital insonation of the carotid siphon. **c** Suboccipital (i.e. transnuchal) insonation of the vertebrobasilar system. For insonation of the distal vertebral artery (*V*) the beam is aimed at the bridge of the nose (*B*). At an insonation depth of approximately 85 mm the junction of the vertebral arteries (*J*) is most often found. This landmark corresponds to the pontile-medullary junction of the brain stem. *T* corresponds to the top of the basilar artery at an insonation depth of approximateley 110 mm. *Numericals 1–3* refer to the various positions of the probe during insonation of the different segments of the vertebrobasilar system

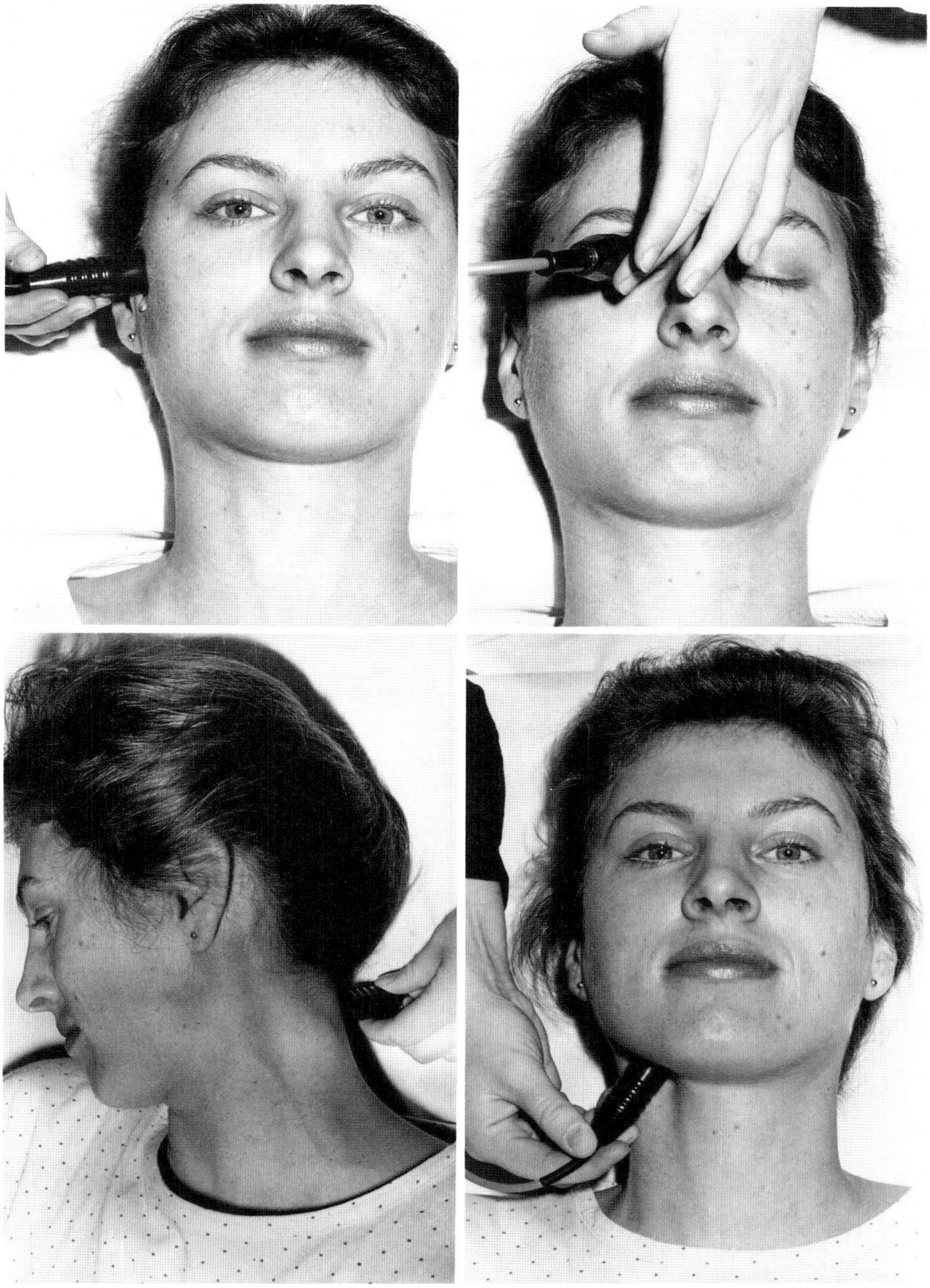

a b c d

Fig. 4a–d. Demonstration of position of the probe during transtemporal (**a**), transorbital (**b**), suboccipital (**c**), and submandibular (**d**) transcranial Doppler sonography

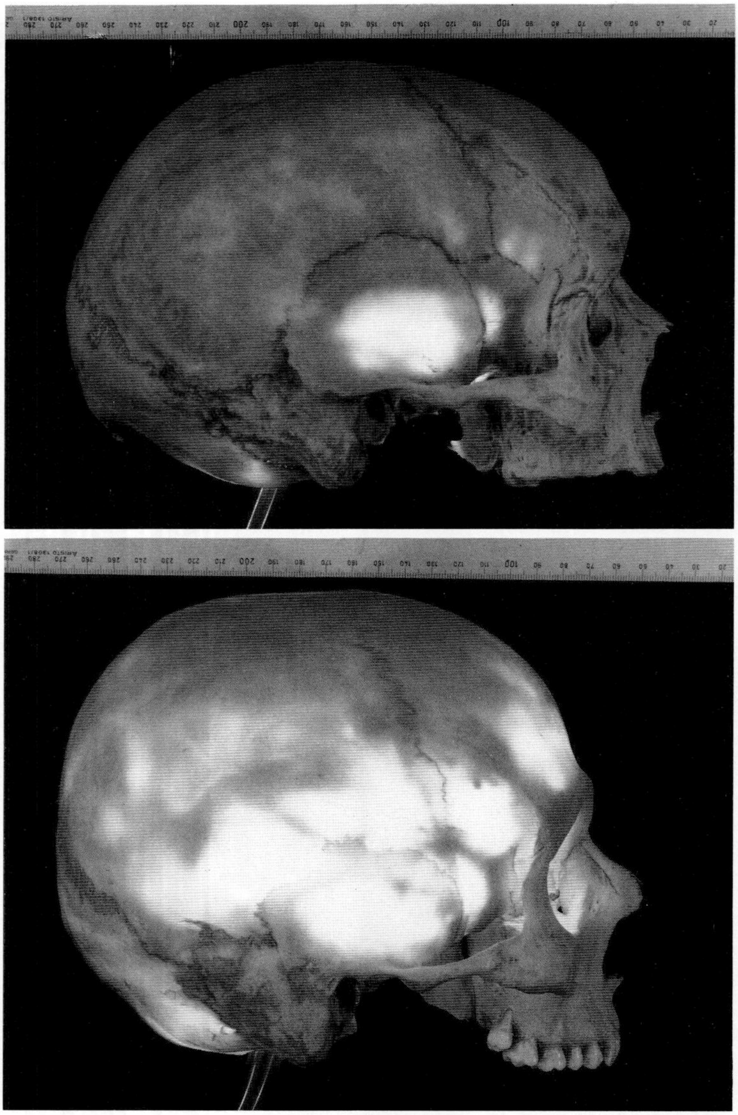

a

b

Fig. 5a, b. Demonstration of the so-called "ultrasound window" in two different skulls. The skulls are illuminated by a standardized light source. A very small (**a**) and a very large (**b**) ultrasound window are demonstrated

Clinical Applications

The list of presently known and clinically useful applications of transcranial Doppler sonography is impressive (Table 2). This list, however, is not complete and is intended only to give an idea of the broad applicability of this new ultrasound tool. The following overview cannot refer in detail to each of these transcranial Doppler ultrasound applications but can focus only on a number of major topics.

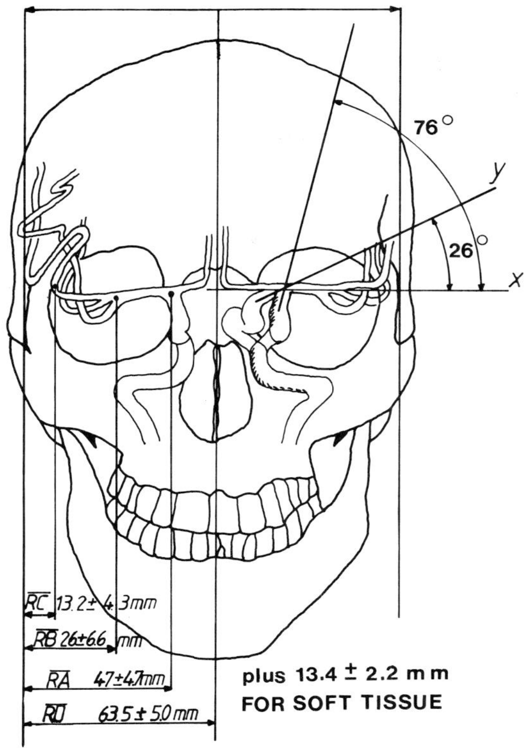

Fig. 6. Demonstration of typical insonation depths in the anterior cerebral circulation. The distances *RC, RB, RA, RD* refer to typical landmarks of the cerebral vasculature as demonstrated during cerebral angiography. The average insonation depths are given. A value of 13.4±2.2 mm must be added for the thickness of the temporal soft tissue. The angle between the M1 segment of the MCA (*X*) and the C1 segment of the ICA (*Y*) varies widely, between 26° and 76° [2]

Diagnosis of Intracranial Cerebrovascular Occlusive Disease

TCD is an important part of a complete noninvasive diagnostic examination of the acute stroke patient. This is shown in the flow chart in Fig. 8. As soon as computerized tomography has been performed and extracranial arterial findings have been evaluated by means of continuous wave Doppler sonography, transcranial Doppler may deliver additional decisive information with reference to both hemodynamic effects of extracranial lesions on intracranial blood flow and detection of intracranial lesions themselves. An example of TCD evaluation of middle cerebral artery stenosis is given in Fig. 9. Figure 9a shows the highly pathologic flow signal in this patient who suffered from fluctuating right-sided hemiplegia and aphasia. Flow signals indicate that flow velocity was abnormally high (>3 Hz, or >120 cm/s) and that a bidirectional, low-frequency enhanced signal appeared during each systole. The latter was indicative of vibrating vessel wall movements and disturbed blood flow. The normal flow signal of the contralateral side is also shown for comparison (Fig. 9b). The diagnosis of a high-grade intracranial MCA stenosis was made but could not be confirmed during selective cerebral angiography. However, insisting on the ultrasound diagnosis, angiography was repeated in further views and, finally, could document the ex-

Table 1. Criteria for identification of various intracranial arterial segments during common carotid artery compression tests

Reaction		Insonated arterial segment	Neuroangiological meaning[1]: configuration of circle of Willis
Any effects of ipsilateral compression test?	If "no":	a) Unsuccessful compression maneuver: try again	
		b) P2	Nonembryonal type of PCA[2]
		c) P1	Absence of posterior collateral pathway[3]
		d) ICA or MCA or A1 or PCoA	Ipsilateral ICA occlusion; clarify extracranial Doppler findings
	If "yes":	Go ahead!	
Decreased flow velocity?	If "yes":	a) MCA	Existence of collateral pathways[4]
		b) PCoA or P2	Embryonal type of PCA; existence of collateral pathways[5]
		c) C1 (ICA)	Existence of posterior collateral pathway
		d) A1	Only existence of posterior collateral pathway
	If "no":	Go ahead!	
Flow inversion?	If "yes":	a) A1 or C1 (ICA)	Existence of internal anterior collateral pathway[6]
		b) PCoA	Existence of posterior collateral pathway
	If "no":	Go ahead!	
Flow stoppage?	If "yes":	a) MCA or C1 (ICA) or A1	Lack of collateral pathways
		b) P2 or PCoA	Embryonal type of PCA; lack of collateral pathways
	If "no":	Go ahead!	
Increased flow velocity?	If "yes":	P1 or PCoA	Existence of posterior collateral pathway
	If "no":	Go ahead!	
Alternating flow?[7]	If "yes":	a) C1 (ICA) or A1	Existence of both anterior and posterior collateral pathways
		b) PCoA	Embryonal type of PCA; existence of both anterior and posterior collateral pathways
	If "no":	Inadequate examination technique: try again	

[1] Provided that
- ICA and CCA are not occluded,
- flow conditions in patients with residual trigeminal artery are not considered,
- retrograde basilar flow in proximal basilar occlusion or manifest steal mechanism is not considered.

[2] Nonembryonal type refers to PCA blood supply exclusively via basilar artery, in contrast to 'embryonal type' indicating partial or complete PCA blood supply via ICA.

[3] This term refers to a collateral pathway from basilar artery via P1 segment of posterior cerebral artery and posterior communicating artery to internal carotid artery.

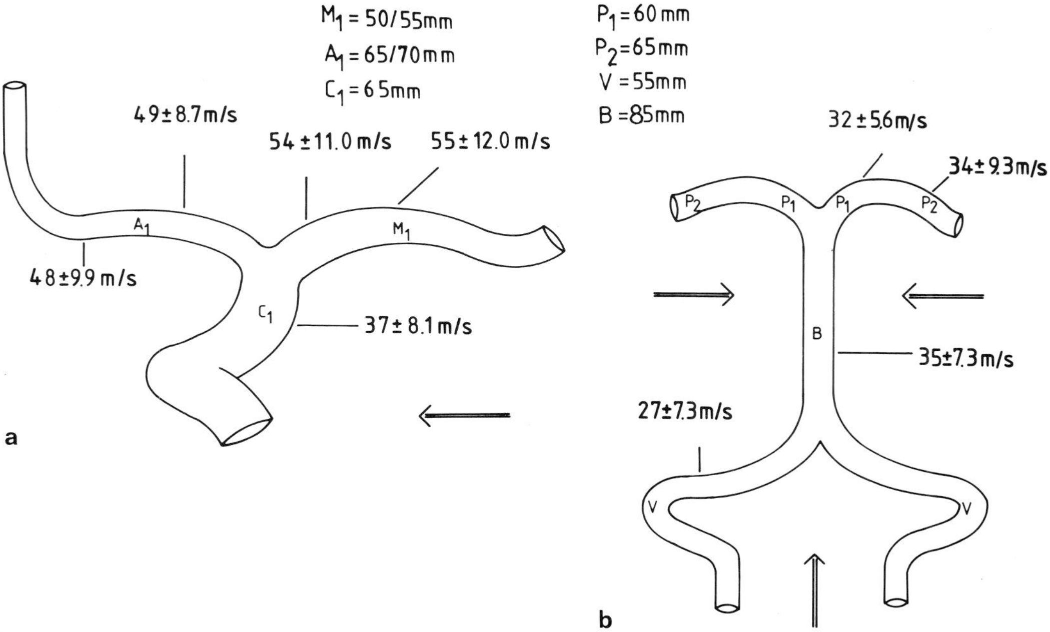

Fig. 7a,b. Normal velocity values within the different cerebral arteries.
a Anterior circulation; **b** posterior circulation. The overall average values for the mean flow velocity within the various vessel segments from 76 normal volunteers are given for the M1 segment of the MCA at insonation depths of 50 and 55 mm, A1 segment of the ACA at insonation depths of 65 and 70 mm, the C1 segment of the carotid siphon at 65 mm, the P1 segment of the posterior cerebral artery at 60 mm, the P2 segment of the posterior cerebral artery at 65 mm, the distal vertebral arteries (V) at 55 mm and the basilar artery (B) at 85 mm insonation depths. The standard deviation is also indicated. *Arrows* indicate propagation of the ultrasound beam

pected subtotal MCA stenosis (Fig. 9c). Similar findings were also available in the posterior circulation during the detection of intracranial vertebral artery stenoses and basilar trunk lesions (Fig. 10).

The comparison of TCD and angiographic findings of a preliminary series of 72 stroke patients (Ringelstein, unpublished data) are summarized in Table 3. Sensitivity and specificity of transcranial Doppler diagnosis when compared with intra-arterial digital subtraction arteriography, as the momentarily best available

---

[4] The precise type of pathway cannot be defined yet.
[5] With the 'pure' embryonal type of PCA blood supply, P2 blood flow indicates existence of both PCoA and anterior collateral pathways in this particular situation.
[6] The term *'internal* anterior cross-filling' refers to cross-flow via the anterior communicating artery to the contralateral MCA territory, in contrast to an *'external* anterior cross-filling' via the external carotid artery to the contralateral ophthalmic artery in cases with both contralateral ICA and ECA occlusion.
[7] This term refers to a regular biphasic change of flow direction during each cardiac circle due to a labile watershed situation.

Table 2. Clinical applications of TCD

1) Diagnosis of intracranial occlusive disease (individual) and epidemiologic aspects
2) Auxiliary test for extracranial occlusive disease (in inconclusive extracranial tests)
3) Evaluation of hemodynamic effects of EOD on intracranial blood flow (ICA occlusion, subclavian steal, etc.)
4) Detection/identification of feeders of AV malformations
5) Preoperative compression tests: What happens intracranially if ...? (analysis of collateralizing capacities of circle of Willis)
6) Intermittent monitoring and follow-up studies
   - of vasospasm in subarachnoid hemorrhage
   - of vasospasm in migraine
   - of spontaneous or therapeutically induced recanalization of occluded vessels
   - after occluding interventions: establishment of collateral pathways, etc.
   - of occlusive disease during anticoagulative therapy
   - of feeders of AV malformations during radiation therapy and other kinds of treatment
   - cerebral flow velocity studies at high altitudes and during acute mountain sideness
   - repetitive examinations for treatment control in sickle cell anomia
7) Continuous monitoring
   - during neuroradiological interventions (balloon occlusion, embolization, etc.)
   - during acute pharmacological trials of vasoactive drugs
   - during carotid endarterectomy (shunt?)
   - during cardiac surgery (ischemic encephalopathy?)
   - during increasing intracranial pressure
   - during evolution of brain death
8) Function tests: Flow velocity measurements
   - during CO_2 stimulation of cerebral vasomotor response
   - during flicker light stimulation of the occipital cortex
9) Noninvasive auxiliary test in animal experiments (nonhuman primate stroke models)

EOD = extracranial occlusive disease
ICA = internal carotid artery

standard, were as high as 87%. Due to the preliminary character of the study, these results may improve with increasing experience of the examiner. Typical pitfalls are listed in Table 4. These refer principally to misinterpretation of high-flow collateral pathways as stenotic lesions, misidentification of the insonated vessel segment, displacement of intracranial arteries due to space-occupying lesions and failures of the angiographic examination to locate exactly the presumed stenotic lesions (Fig. 9). It can be expected that these pitfalls may gradually be reduced with increasing experience.

Table 3. Sensitivity and specificity of TCD for the detection of intracranial CVD (n = 72)

Standard: selective intra-arterial DSA
Prevalence: 32/72 = 44%

		TCD		
		+	–	
Intra-arterial DSA	+	28	4	Sens. = 0.875
	–	5	35	Spec. = 0.875

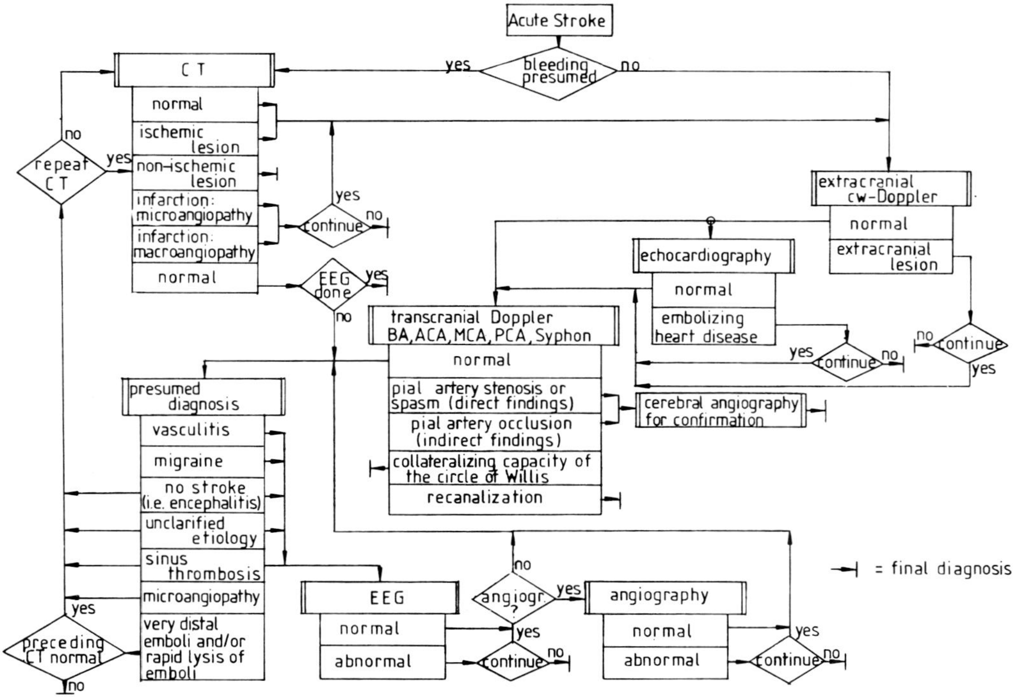

Fig. 8. Flow chart of the diagnostic procedure in patients with acute stroke. After CCT and extracranial CW Doppler studies a transcranial examination, echocardiography, laboratory tests and EEG are performed in order to clarify the pathogenesis of the stroke. If necessary a repeated CCT and, as a last step, angiography are also conducted. In normal extracranial CW Doppler findings TCD should be performed in order to identify an intracranial lesion of the large basal cerebral arteries. In severe extracranial occlusive disease TCD examination can deliver further information about their hemodynamic effects on intracranial blood flow

Table 4. Typical errors and failures in use of TCD

1. Arterial lesion not within the resolution of TCD (e.g. distal branch occlusion)	3[a]
2. Collateral PCoA-flow misinterpreted as siphon "stenosis"	3
3. Failure of unknown reason; lesions not detected by TCD	2
4. Vertebrobasilar collateral channel misinterpreted as vertebral stenosis	1
5. Stenosis of A1-segment not detected	1
6. Hemorrhage-induced displacement of MCA misinterpreted as MCA occlusion	1
7. C4-stenosis not detected ("relative blind spot")	1
8. Failure of initial angiogram to demonstrate lesion	3[a]

[a] Counted as correct TCD diagnoses

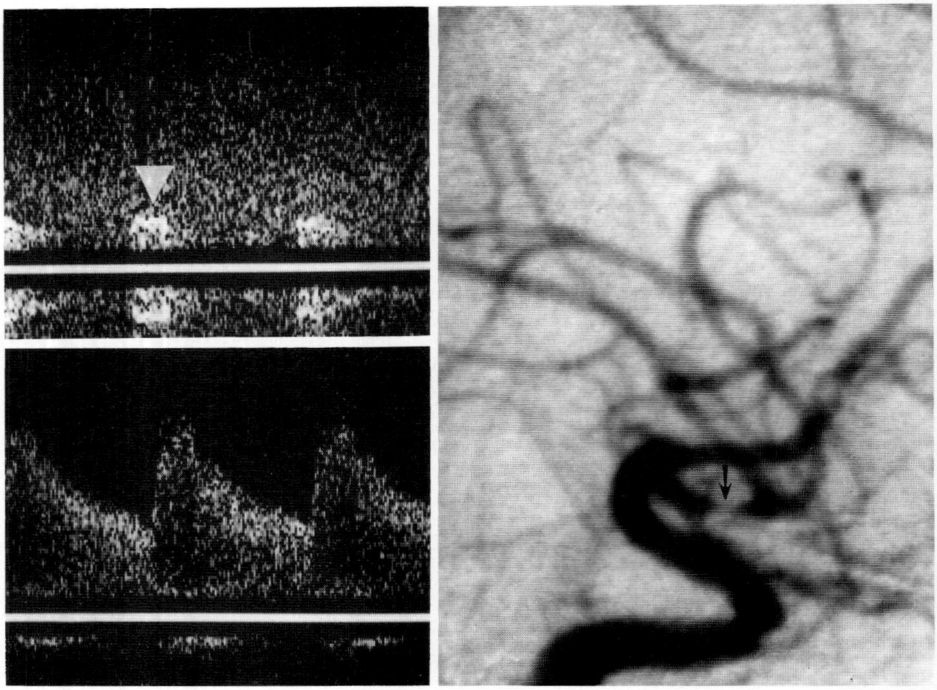

a b c

Fig. 9 a – c. Subtotal middle cerebral artery stenosis in a middle-aged man with fluctuating aphasia and hemiplegia.
a Transcranical Doppler sonography on the left side revealed severely increased flow velocity within the M1 segment of the MCA, turbulent blood flow, vessel wall vibration phenomena and a faint musical murmur (*arrowhead*). **b** The normal flow signal of the contralateral MCA at the same insonation depth is also demonstrated (for calibration see Fig. 11). **c** After the initial intra-arterial digital subtraction angiography has been found to be normal; a second angiography in a more oblique view clearly indicated the subtotal MCA stenosis (*arrow*). Heparin therapy led to prompt relief from ischemic attacks

Hemodynamic Effects of Extracranial Lesions on Cerebral Blood Flow

In the vertebrobasilar system the subclavian steal mechanism serves as a model. During suboccipital insonation, the *feeding* vertebral artery, the *stealing* vertebral artery and the *basilar* trunk can be differentiated from each other by means of their blood-flow characteristics, particularly during brachial hyperemia [5]. An

Fig. 10 a – c. Transcranial Doppler diagnosis of a vertebrobasilar stenosis.
a At an insonation depth of 65 mm a high-velocity flow signal with turbulent flow was found and was attributed to the right distal vertebral or posterior inferior cerebellar artery, respectively. A more precise topographical diagnosis was not possible. **a** At the same insonation depth a quite normal flow signal was also found in the vicinity and was erroneously attributed to the left distal vertebral artery. **c** Angiography, however, showed a hypertrophic posterior inferior cerebellar artery (*arrow*) and a long stenotic segment of the left distal vertebral artery (*double arrow*). The patient suffered from fluctuating brainstem symptoms. Heparin therapy prompted cessation of symptoms

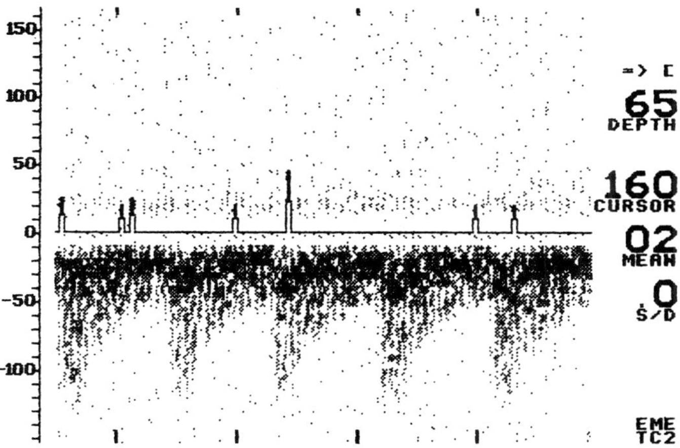
150
100
50
0
-50
-100
=> [
65
DEPTH
160
CURSOR
02
MEAN
.0
S/D
EME
TC2
a

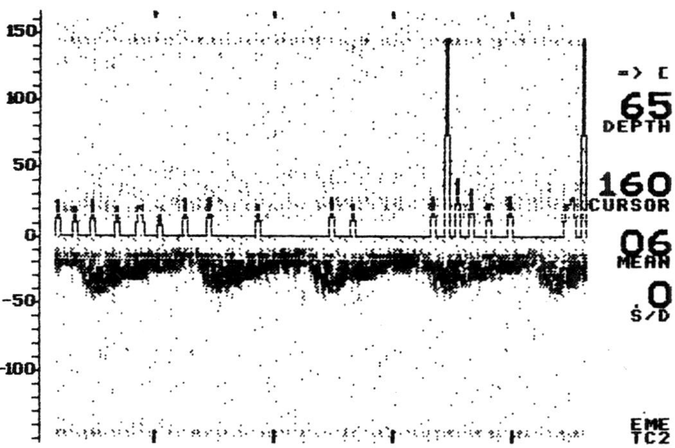
150
100
50
0
-50
-100
=> [
65
DEPTH
160
CURSOR
06
MEAN
.0
S/D
EME
TC2
b

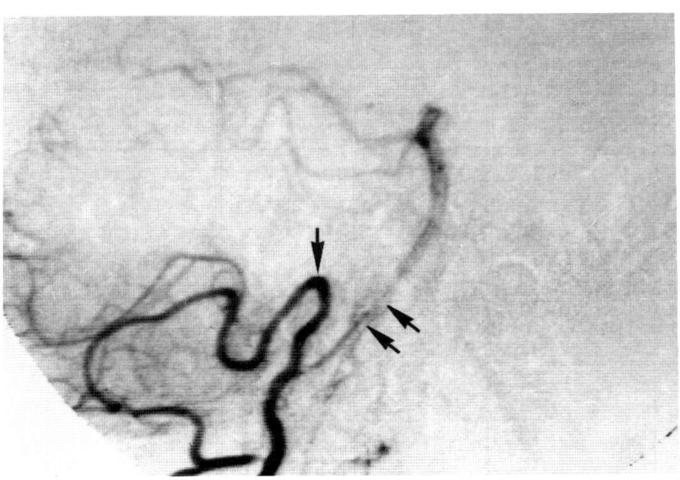
c

example is presented in Fig. 11. The findings indicate that under special conditions, basilar artery blood flow velocity may be affected more or less severely by extracranial occlusive disease of the proximal subclavian artery. However, this is a relatively rare event. In a series of 91 patients with various degrees of subclavian steal, only 13 showed severe disturbances of basilar artery blood flow, namely either alternating blood flow during brachial hyperemia or even flow reversal during the whole cardiac cycle [5]. It should be noted that such severe flow disturbances occurred only in patients with bilateral subclavian vertebral artery lesions and not in a merely unilateral subclavian artery stenosis or occlusion.

Figure 11 depicts the findings in an extreme case with a right-sided subclavian artery occlusion, left-sided subtotal subclavian artery stenosis and proximal common carotid artery stenosis on the left. When at rest, this patient had severe basilar artery flow disturbances with a dampened orthograde flow signal during systole and reversal of the blood column during diastole. The net flow was virtually nil. Brachial hyperemia on the left side led to an immediate complete reversal of basilar artery blood flow (not shown here) with an accentuation of her complaint. She then had spells of vertigo and double vision. Subsequently, this patient was subjected to percutaneous transluminal angioplasty of the left proximal subclavian artery via a transfemoral route inducing abolishment of the steal mechanism and normal blood flow to the arm. A moderate stenosis of the origin of the vertebral artery became apparent (Fig. 11c). Considerable improvement in blood flow within the basilar trunk and stable basilar artery flow despite provocative tests on the brachial arteries could be established (Fig. 11d). Further aspects of the influence of extracranial lesion within the carotid system on intracranial blood flow are detailed later, in the section referring to curtailment of the cerebral vasomotor response.

Transcranial Doppler Monitoring

The first application of TCD for monitoring purposes was the intermittent reexamination of flow velocities within the basal arteries of patients after subarachnoid hemorrhage who were presumed to suffer from *hemorrhage-induced vasospasm*. Systematic studies in this field by Aaslid et al. [6, 7], Harders [8], and Seiler et al. [9] have shown that increased flow velocity and spasm closely correlate in the expected direction with the following:

1. Both the size and extention of the blood clot
2. The clinical state of the patient according to the Hunt and Hess scale [10]
3. The angiographically visualized severity of the spasm (if flow velocity >3 KHz, or 120 cm/s)
4. The side of the predominant location of the blood clot and, thus, the presumed site of the aneurysm (this also corresponds to the side of the operative approach)
5. A further very important parameter for the patient's prognosis has shown itself to be the increase in blood flow velocity within the first few days after acute bleeding, i.e. between day 4 and day 10. A sharp increase indicates a markedly worse prognosis.

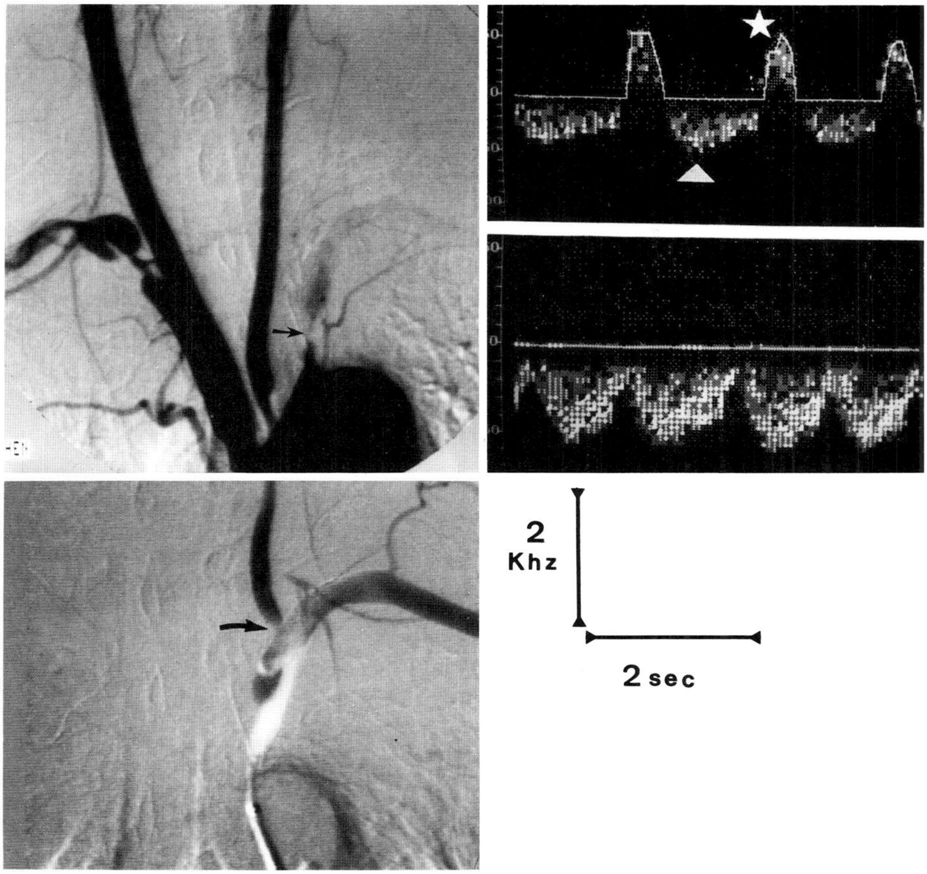

a b c

Fig. 11a–d. Basilar artery flow disturbances due to severe subclavian steal mechanism. **a** Angiography confirmed the extracranial Doppler findings and showed a proximal stenosis, as well as distal occlusion of the right subclavian artery, a proximal stenosis of the left common carotid artery and a subtotal stenosis of the left subclavian artery (*arrow*). **b** Due to the severe extracranial disease, blood flow within the basilar trunk was alternating with a dampened flow signal in the cephalad direction during systole (*arrowhead*) and a high resistance flow signal in the retrograde direction during diastole (*asterix*). **c** After successful percutaneous transluminal angioplasty of the left-side subclavian artery stenosis, blood flow to the left axillary artery became normal. A slight stenosis at the orifice of the left vertebral artery became visible (*arrow*). **d** Angioplasty led to a nearly normal and orthograde blood flow within the basilar trunk. (Downward-deflected curve means cephalad blood flow direction within the basilar artery and vice versa)

"Critical" flow velocities due to vasospasm within the MCA were found to be 3 KHz Doppler shift, which corresponds to 120 cm/s. "Highly critical" spasm with a considerable probability of producing brain infarctions was associated with flow velocities of 3.5 KHz Doppler shift or even more. The typical 4-week time course after the initial bleeding was characterized by an initial increase of flow velocity and then a gradual decrease after an approximately 10-day plateau. Spasm-induced high flow velocities of the MCA were modulated in the expected direction by application of calcium antagonists (decrease), and by performance of cerebral angiography during the spasm phase (increase). An example of the development of severe vasospasm with subsequent cerebral infarction, brain swelling and resulting brain death is demonstrated in Fig. 12.

Continuous intraoperative *monitoring of middle cerebral artery blood flow velocity during carotid endarterectomy* is another exciting field of TCD application. From our limited experiences and from those of others [11, 12, 13] this new approach promises help in a number of ways. (a) Preoperatively it can be used to predict the collateralizing capacities of the circle of Willis and the need for intraoperative shunting. (b) It is also interesting to study the relationship between systemic arterial blood pressure and MCA flow velocity during carotid endarterectomy both when the artery is clamped and when it is reflooded. (c) It would also be of interest for vascular surgeons in comparing MCA flow velocity measurements with other parameters of intracranial collateralization, such as carotid artery stump pressure and intensity of backbleeding. (d) In particular cases it may offer help to the vascular surgeon in assessing whether a shunt function is adequate. (e) TCD can also teach us the kinds of effects which can be expected on MCA blood flow velocity from removal of stenotic internal carotid artery lesions of various degrees of severity. This is particularly true for patients with bilateral ICA obstructions or multifocal occlusive disease of the extracranial brain-supplying arteries. (f) The most important aspect in our own view, however, lies in correlating MCA flow changes with electrical functions of the depleted MCA territory by means of electrophysiological parameters. This would perhaps allow us to define a lowest tolerable and safe MCA flow velocity which is necessary to guarantee functional integrity of the brain. TCD monitoring of 64 patients during carotid endarterectomy and cross-clamping without a shunt has revealed that intraoperative blockage of the carotid arteries is by far more frequently tolerated without any cerebral hazards than had previously been thought [13]. This means that an intraoperative shunt is generally too often used. The shunt, however, has its own intrinsic morbidity by subjecting the patient to the risk of plaque or thrombus embolization and dissection.

A comparably new and promising approach is TCD monitoring of both MCA flow velocity and air-bubble passage during *open heart surgery* [14, 15]. This has already led to new insights into the pathophysiology of postoperative encephalopathy following cardiopulmonary bypass.

In rare cases, transcranial Doppler sonography may deliver decisive information for *interventional neuroradiologic procedures*, both recanalizing and occluding. Recently we have published the case of an 18-year-old boy with a inoperable but progressively symptomatic giant aneurysm of the basilar artery. After application of three occluding balloons within both vertebral arteries and one major collateral pathway, it was possible to reduce flow velocity dramatically within the proximal basilar trunk. This, finally, led to spontaneous thrombosis of the aneurysm. The complex and risky sequence of interventions during this type of treatment could be advocated only after each particular vessel occlusion had been proven to be safe with respect to brainstem ischemia. Preinterventional compression tests under simultaneous basilar artery transcranial Doppler and evoked potential monitoring were used and, obviously, induced adequate therapeutic

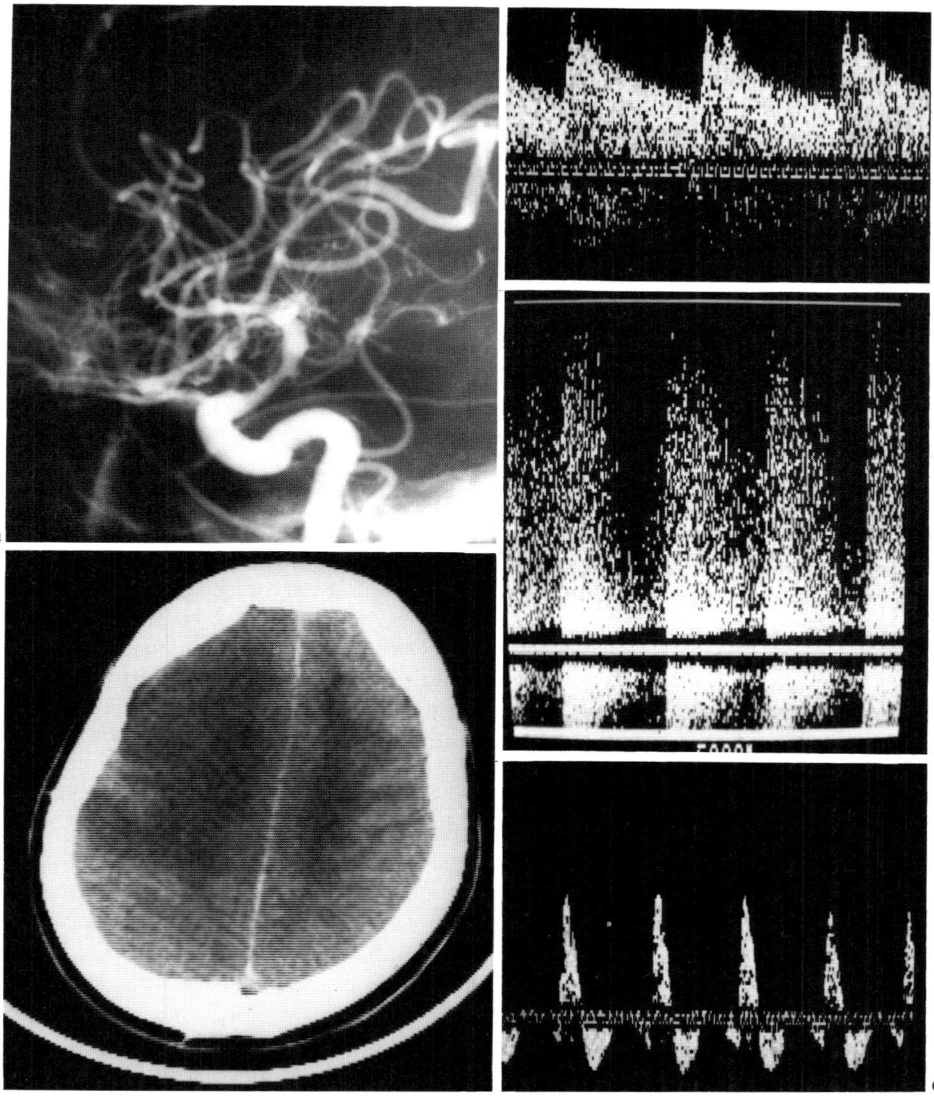

Fig. 12a–e. Subarachnoid hemorrhage from a berry aneurysm with subsequent vasospasm, cerebral infarction and brain death.

a Angiography demonstrated severe vasospasm in several supraclinoidal vessel segments. **b** Initially, flow velocity was normal within the MCA. **c** After several days, however, vasospasm led to a dramatic increase in flow velocity and severe turbulences. The latter was indicated by the symmetrical low frequency signals during systole. **d** Severe vasospasm led to bilateral brain infarctions. **e** Due to uncontrollable brain swelling, circulatory arrest within the cerebral arteries occurred and led to a pendulum-like, so-called "reverberating," flow within the large intracranial arteries, due to stoppage of blood flow in the peripheral vascular network. As soon as this flow signal appeared, all clinical signs of brain death occurred [11]. For calibration see Fig. 11

decisions in this endangered patient. The treatment was completely successful [16].

In animal experiments with primates TCD may also provide valuable information during artificial MCA occlusions and other flow-reducing procedures.

These examples should suffice to give an impression of the potential usefulness of transcranial Doppler sonography as a monitoring instrument in clinical and scientific settings.

Vasomotor Response of Cerebral Vasculature

Doppler techniques are highly sensitive for online registration of even minor flow velocity changes, particularly in hemodynamically labile situations. In contrast to the injection of contrast medium during cerebral angiography, ultrasound does not intervene with the natural hemodynamic conditions, i.e., artifacts induced by the procedure itself can be avoided.

One of the most attractive concepts in stroke research is the existence of ischemic penumbra preceding definite ischemic tissue damage. This means that after manifestation of brain ischemia a short but definite period remains for therapeutic measures to prevent complete tissue damage [17].

Gibbs et al. [18] have demonstrated that an increased oxygen extraction rate from the blood is indicative of true ischemia. In this case, the compensatory mechanism of vessel dilatation (vasomotor reserve) is nearly or already exhausted. It is known that during maximal dilatation of the resistance vessels in order to counterbalance a critical drop of perfusion pressure, the cerebral arterioles are also no longer able to react to CO_2 stimuli. This is why cerebral CO_2-induced vasomotor reactivity can be used as an indicator of a more or less exhausted vasomotor reserve. Arterial territories can be identified which show a truly critical and insufficiently compensated drop of perfusion pressure. The functional state of the vasomotors is mirrored by the flow velocity within the MCA artery [19]. This is demonstrated in Fig. 13. When the vasomotors are dilated due to CO_2 stimulation, flow velocity within the MCA stem increases, whereas during hypocapnia MCA flow velocity is reduced. During transcranial Doppler studies of the MCA flow velocity, the above-mentioned relation may be used to measure the actual state of vasomotor reactivity within the MCA territory. In normal subjects and in those with (a) stepwise decreasing hypercapnia (i.e., 5%, 4%, 3%, 2% CO_2 content of air), (b) normocapnia (i.e., breathing of room air), and (c) stepwise increasing hypercapnia due to hyperventilation, the relative changes of flow velocity within the MCA stem can be measured [20]. These values were plotted against the end tidal CO_2 values of the patient. In volunteers of different age and sex, changes in MCA flow velocity of approximately $100 \pm 15\%$ were found to be normal. In patients with severe reduction of perfusion pressure, however, e.g., those with unilateral or bilateral ICA occlusion, CO_2-induced vasomotor reactivity of the ipsilateral MCA territory may be reduced to zero or even negative values. An example is given in Fig. 14. In a preliminary series of 12 chronic patients with unilateral ICA occlusion and 8 chronic patients with bilateral ICA occlusions, however, only one patient in the former group and two in the latter showed a severe curtailment of vasomotor reactivity to less than 33%. These three were

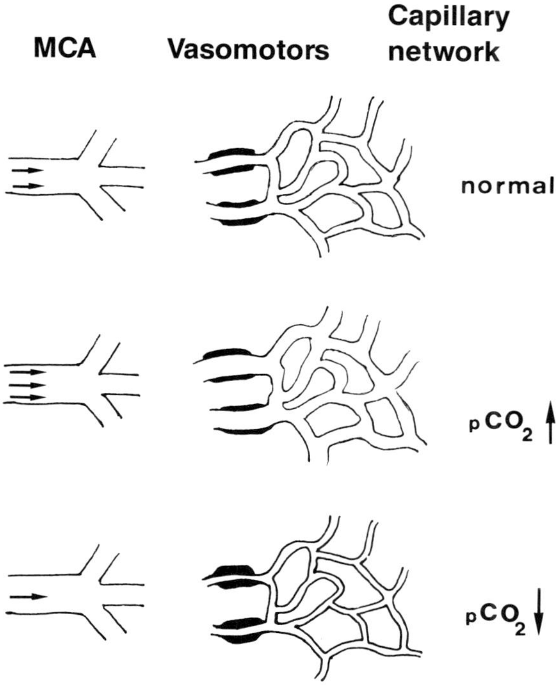

Fig. 13. Influence of the functional state of the cerebral vasomotor arteries on middle cerebral artery blood flow velocity. *Upper:* Normal flow conditions. *Middle:* Due to a CO_2-induced vasodilation flow velocity within the MCA trunk increases. The contrary is the case during hypocapnia due to hyperventilation (*lower*). MCA = middle cerebral artery. (From [19])

symptomatic, presenting either hypostatic TIAs [21] or progressive ischemic ophthalmopathy [22]. Obviously, the severe degree of vasomotor reactivity reduction in these cases was critical and led to functional disturbances of the neural tissue and chronic progressive damage of the retina.

Another series of five patients was subjected to CO_2-dependent vasomotor reactivity measurements before and after endarterectomy of high-grade ICA stenoses. These findings also indicated that hemodynamically significant ICA lesions can severely affect and even exhaust the compensatory capacities of the vasomotor system. Whereas preoperative VMR was strikingly reduced in these patients on the affected side, postoperative measurements revealed nearly complete normalization of this parameter. These findings show that transcranial Doppler sonography may be used as a noninvasive tool to evaluate the compensatory state of the cerebral vasculature under normal and pathologic conditions. It may also be helpful to define the hemodynamic impact of high-grade ICA stenoses and to select candidates for prophylactic endarterectomy [23].

The *conclusions* drawn from these studies were twofold. (a) Even bilateral ICA occlusions do not necessarily lead to severe hemodynamic disturbances within the MCA territories. Obviously, the compensatory capacities of the cerebral vascular tree to counterbalance severe perfusion pressure reduction is generally underestimated. This may, at least in part, explain unsatisfactory therapeutic results of theoretically beneficial recanalizing procedures, such as ECIC bypassing. (b) The transcranial Doppler evaluation of the vasomotor reac-

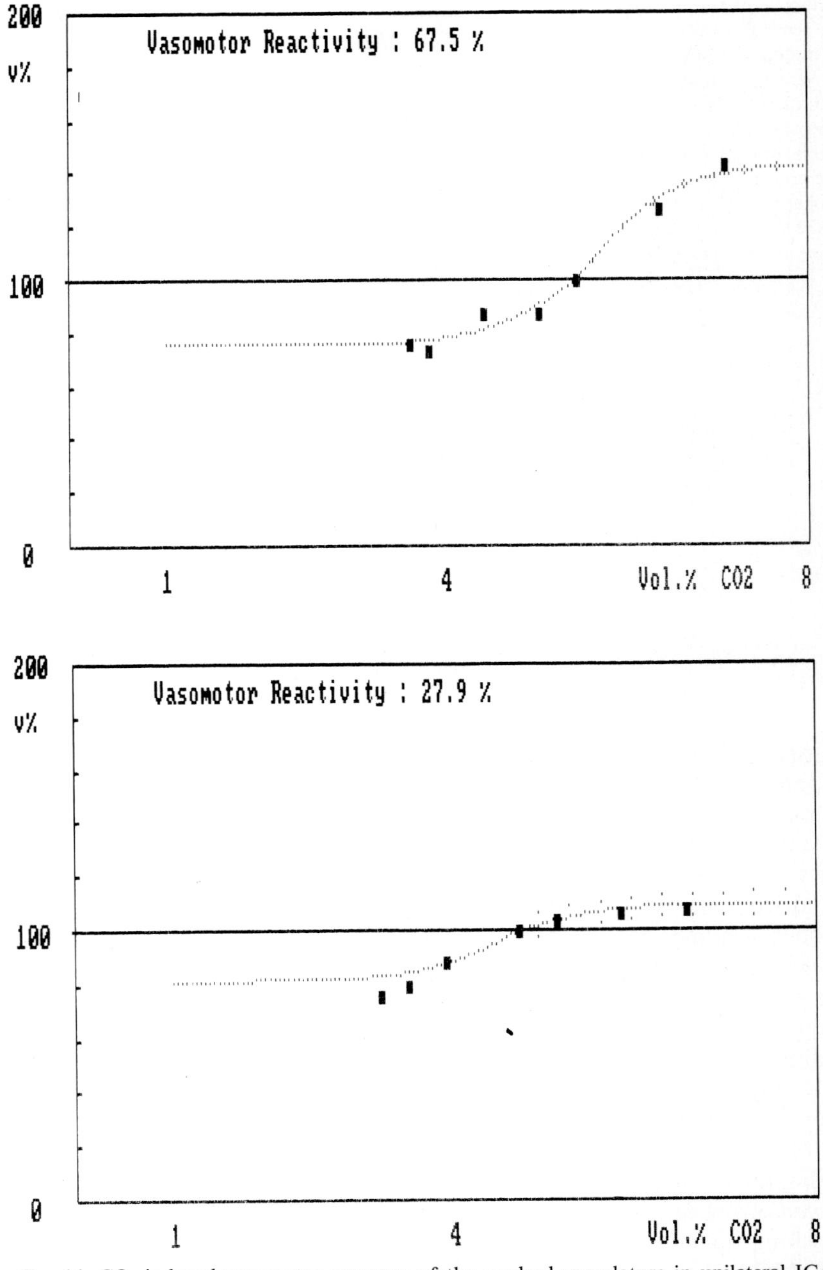

Fig. 14. CO_2-induced vasomotor response of the cerebral vasculature in unilateral ICA occlusion. *Upper,* the bi-asymptotic curve indicates a slightly reduced modulation of blood flow velocity within the MCA stem during hyper- and hypocapnia of 67.5% (normal range 88 ± 15%). This value was measured on the nonaffected side. *Lower,* on the occluded side, due to lack of collateralizing pathways, vasomotor reactivity was dramatically reduced to 27.9%. This patient suffered from ischemic ophthalmopathy. (V% = changes of flow velocity at rest in percent)

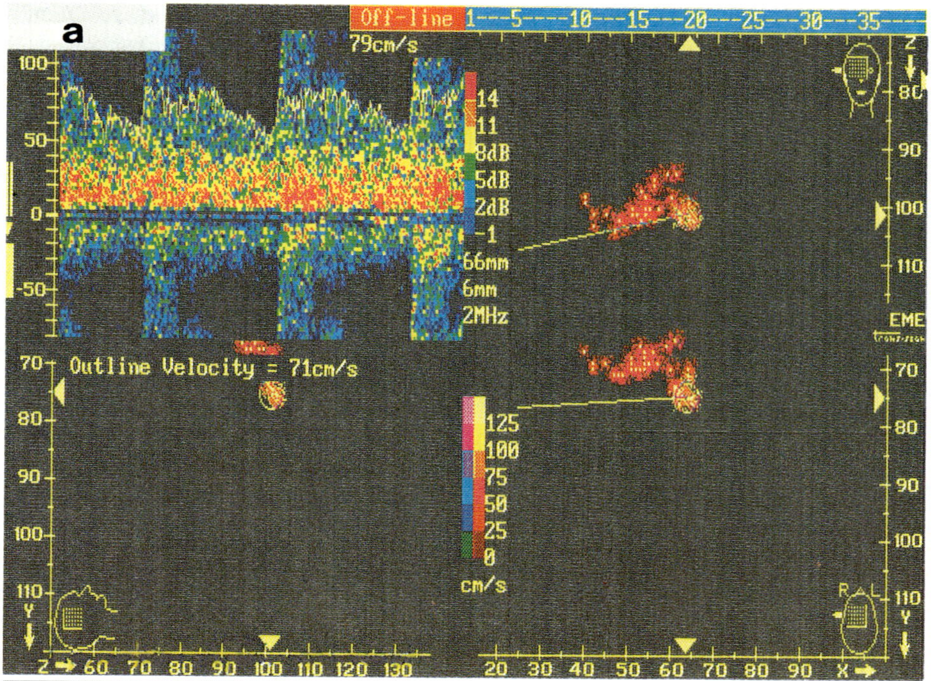

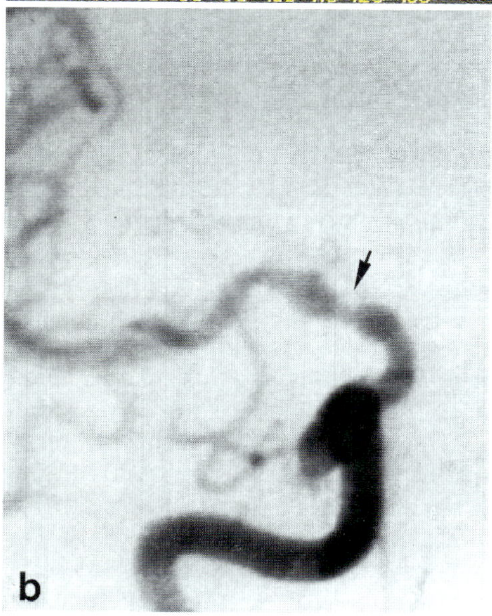

Fig. 15 a, b. Flow mapping of the circle of Willis and adjacent brain-supplying arteries in a patient with right-sided siphon stenosis within the C1 segment.
a The stenotic area is indicated by abnormally high flow velocities and turbulent blood flow (see *yellow dots* where sample volume is placed on the right). The flow signals are shown on the *left*. The cerebral vasculature is reconstructed in the frontal (*upper right*), and axial (*lower right*) plane. **b** Angiography revealed the expected medium-sized C1 stenosis (*arrow*)

tivity of cerebral vessels may be used as a very sensitive instrument to identify these rare cases in which vasomotor reserve is critically reduced. It is hypothesized that this very small subgroup of patients contains the candidates that theoretically might benefit from operative recanalization or vascular microsurgery.

Not only the operative recanalization of a large cerebral artery but also the improvement of the *rheological blood properties* may influence the reactivity span of the cerebral vasomotors during CO_2 stimulation. In a previous paper [24] we have reported on a severe reduction of CO_2-induced vasomotor reactivity in patients with hyperviscosity syndrome due to severe paraproteinemia. After plasmapheresis, however, a dramatic normalization of the vasomotor reactivity could be demonstrated. Comparable effects could be found in patients suffering from subcortical arteriosclerotic encephalopathy (SAE) of the Binswanger type [24]. Initially, most of the patients had a clearly abnormal vasomotor reactivity when compared to age-matched healthy volunteers. In a trial, plasma hyperviscosity of these patients was reduced by a 4-week subcutaneous application of ancrod. The resulting drop in plasma viscosity was paralleled by a significant increase and normalization of CO_2-induced vasomotor reactivity. However, in the SAE patients, it could not be demonstrated that this improvement of flow conditions lead to any beneficial clinical effect [25].

Conclusions and Further Perspectives

Transcranial Doppler sonography is a new noninvasive neuroangiological instrument with truly promising perspectives in its clinical application. Presently, this technique is ideal for noninvasive surveillance and evaluation of hemodynamic alterations of cerebral blood flow within the basal cerebral arteries. With some training the examination technique is relatively easy to learn for monitoring purposes. By contrast, a topographically and quantitatively precise diagnosis of intracranial occlusive processes is still a delicate procedure. Identification of stenoses, occlusions and collateral pathways requires a very time-consuming examination technique and substantial personal expertise to make correct diagnoses. Some of these difficulties will hopefully be overcome with the help of a new transcranial Doppler imaging system, the so-called brain mapping. This technique aims at reconstructing the configuration of the basal vascular tree. This is done with the help of a helmet-like guideway for the probes on either side. Manipulations of the sample volume are transferred to a coordinate system and both flow velocity and flow direction are displayed as colour-coded dots. An example from our laboratory is shown in Fig. 15 from a middle-aged man with right-sided siphon stenosis (C1 segment). The mapping system is particularly useful for an anatomically correct identification of the placement of the sample volume and for rapid reorientation within the network of the brain vasculature, as well as for a multimodal objective documentation of the findings for off-line diagnosis.

Acknowledgements. The author is greatly indebted to Mrs. Christiane Goebel, Gabi Tietz and Dr. Andreas Holling for technical and artwork assistance, as well as to Mrs. Kati Seidel for secretarial work.

References

1. Aaslid R, Markwalder T-M, Nornes H (1982) Noninvasive transcranial Doppler ultrasound recording of flow velocity in basal cerebral arteries. J Neurosurg 75:769–774
2. Ringelstein EB, Otis SM, Kahlscheuer B, Niggemeyer E (1987) Transcranial Doppler sonography. Part I: Anatomical landmarks and normal velocity values. Submitted for publication
3. Ringelstein EB, Otis SM, Kahlscheuer B, Niggemeyer (1987) Transcranial Doppler sonography. Part II: Examination techniques. Submitted for publication
4. Arnolds BJ, von Reutern G-M (1986) Transcranial Doppler sonography. Examination technique and normal reference values. Ultrasound Med Biol 12:115–123
5. Ringelstein EB, Busker M, Buchner H (1987) Evaluation of hemodynamic effects of subclavian steal mechanisms on basilar artery blood flow with the help of transcranial Doppler sonography. In: Aaslid R, Fieschi C, Zanette EM (eds): Advances in transcranial Doppler sonography. Springer, Vienna New York
6. Aaslid R, Nornes H (1984) Musical murmurs in human cerebral arteries after subarachnoid hemorrhage. J Neurosurg 60:32–36
7. Aaslid R, Huber P, Nornes H (1984) Evaluation of cerebrovascular spasm with transcranial Doppler ultrasound. J Neurosurg 60:37–41
8. Harders A (1986) Monitoring of hemodynamic changes related to vasospasm in the circle of Willis after aneurysm surgery. In: Aaslid R (ed) Transcranial Doppler sonography. Springer, Vienna New York, pp 132–146
9. Seiler RW, Grolimund P, Aaslid R, Huber P, Nornes H (1986) Relation of cerebral vasospasm evaluated by transcranial Doppler ultrasound to clinical grade and CT-visualized subarachnoid hemorrhage. J Neurosurg 64:594–600
10. Hunt WE, Hess RM (1968) Surgical risk as related to time of intervention in the repair of intracranial aneurysms. J Neurosurg 28:14–20
11. Ringelstein EB, Richert F, Bardos S, Minale C, Alsukun M, Zeplin H, Schöndube F, Zeumer H, Messmer B (1985) Transkraniell-sonographisches Monitoring des Blutflusses der A. cerebri media während rekanalisierender Operationen an der extrakraniellen A. carotis interna. Nervenarzt 56:423–430
12. Ringelstein EB (1986) Transcranial Doppler monitoring. In: Aaslid R (ed) Transcranial Doppler sonography. Springer, Vienna New York, pp 147–163
13. Edelmann M, Nielen C, Richert F, Skondras S, Ringelstein EB (1987) TCD monitoring of middle cerebral artery blood flow velocity during carotid endarterectomy. Further experiences. In: Aaslid R, Fieschi C, Zanette EM (eds) Advances in transcranial Doppler sonography. Springer, Vienna New York (in press)
14. Ries F, Eicke M, Murday H, Kirchhoff PG (1987) TCD-monitoring of changes in intracerebral hemodynamics during open heart surgery: correlation to post-operative complications. In: Aaslid R, Fieschi C, Zanette EM (eds) Advances in transcranial Doppler sonography. Springer, Vienna New York (in press)
15. Padayachee TS, Parsons S, Deverall PB, Gosling RG (1987) Detection of microemboli in the middle cerebral artery during cardiopulmonary bypass: a TCD study. In: Aaslid R, Fieschi C, Zanette EM (eds) Advances in transcranial Doppler sonography. Springer, Vienna New York (in press)
16. Ringelstein EB, Wulfinghoff F, Brückmann H, Zeumer H, Hacke W, Buchner H (1985) Transcranial Doppler sonography as a non-invasive guide for the transvascular treatment of an inoperable basilar-artery aneurysm. Neurol Res 7:171–176
17. Astrup J, Siesjö BK, Symon L (1981) Threshold in cerebral ischemia – the ischemic penumbra. Stroke 12:723–725
18. Gibbs JG, Wise RJS, Leeners KL, Jones T (1984) Evaluation of cerebral perfusion reserve in patients with carotid artery occlusion. Lancet 1:182–186, 310–314
19. Ringelstein EB, Otis SM, Grosse W (1987) TCD assessment of carbon dioxide induced vasomotor reactivity in normals and in patients with cerebrovascular disease. In: Aaslid R, Fieschi C, Zanette EM (eds) Advances in transcranial Doppler sonography. Springer, Vienna New York (in press)
20. Kirkham FJ, Padayachee CS, Parsons S, Seargeant LS, House FR, Gosling RG (1986) Transcranial measurement of blood velocities in the basal cerebral arteries using pulsed Doppler ultrasound: velocity as an index of flow. Ultrasound Med Biol 12:5–14

21. Caplan LR, Sergay S (1976) Positional cerebral ischemia. J Neurol Neurosurg Psychiat 39:385–391
22. Carter JE (1985) Chronic ocular ischemia and carotid vascular disease. Stroke 16:721–728
23. Widder B, Paulat K, Hackspacher J, Mayr E (1986) Transcranical Doppler CO_2-test for the detection of hemodynamically critical carotid artery stenoses and occlusions. Eur Arch Psychiatr Neurol Sci 236:162–168
24. Ringelstein EB, Grosse W, Mauckner A, Schneider R, Glöckner WM, Matentzoglu S (1987) Does blood rheology influence vasomotors? A transcranial Doppler study during hypo- and hypercapnia. In: Hartmann A, Kuschinsky W (eds) Cerebral ischemia and hemorheology. Springer, Berlin Heidelberg New York (in press)
25. Ringelstein EB, Mauckner A, Sturm W, Eschenfelder V, Grosse W, Matentzoglu S, Zeumer H, Doering W, Wolf S, Schneider R, Maurin N, Willmes K, Schlenker W (1987) Failure of enzymatic defibrination to improve subcortical arteriosclerotic encephalopathy in an acute trial. In: Cervos-Navarro J, Ferszt R (eds) Pathology of cerebrospinal microcirculation. Raven, New York (in press)
26. Ringelstein EB, Wulfinghoff F (1985) Diagnostische Möglichkeiten der transkraniellen Dopplersonographie in der Neurologie. Angio 7:167–182

Indium-111 Platelet-Scintigraphy in Stroke Patients

C. KESSLER [1]

Introduction

In 1976 Thakur et al. [47] succeeded in labelling human platelets with an indium-111 8-hydroxychinoline complex (oxine). In the beginning, ^{111}In-labelled platelets were used in hematologic disorders to estimate the platelet life span and the site of platelet destruction, e.g., in Werlhof's disease [22, 34]. Since ^{111}In is a gamma-emitting isotope, the recording of gamma-camera images became possible, thereby making visible the incorporation of radiolabelled platelets in thrombus formations.

The increase in therapeutic possibilities for the management of patients with thromboembolic complications, e.g., by fibronolytic treatment or vascular surgery, required further information as to the extent, age, and activity of the thromboembolic material causing clinical symptoms. This information could not be obtained by conventional imaging methods using contrast media or ultrasound techniques. Since the introduction of radiolabelling of autologous platelets with ^{111}In, platelet scintigraphy (PSC) has been used as a diagnostic tool in various thromboembolic diseases. It has a very high specificity in diagnosing deep venous thrombosis [19, 50]. It can be used in imaging pulmonary emboli [5] as well as cardiac thrombi [15, 46] and thrombotic material in abdominal aneurysms [41]. Platelet scintigraphy has also been successful in imaging atherosclerotic lesions in peripheral arteries [16] as well as in coronary [10] and carotid arteries [8, 26]. Several reports have proven that platelet scintigraphy also permits evaluation of the thrombogenicity of vascular grafts [17, 46] and valvular prostheses [12].

Previous attempts at thrombus scintigraphy in vivo using radiolabelled fibrinogen or isotopes other than ^{111}In have, for the most part, remained unsuccessful. Scintigraphy with iodinated fibrinogen failed due to its unspecific binding to the vessel wall [49]. Platelet labelling has also been attempted with ^{99m}Tc. The 6-h half-life of this isotope was, however, too short for measuring the platelet incorporation into thrombi. ^{51}Cr has for years been the most favourable ligand used in platelet labelling and has frequently been used in platelet life-span studies [1]. The low gamma photon emission of ^{51}Cr, however, does not allow the production of scintigraphic images, and its long half-life (27 days) brings the patient an increased exposure to radiation.

^{111}In has proven to be the most useful isotope in platelet labelling. Since it is a lipophilic complex when associated with oxine [42], acetylacetone [43] or

[1] Department of Neurology, Krankenhaus Merheim, Ostmerheimerstr. 200, D-5000 Köln 91, FRG

tropolone [7, 11], ^{111}In is capable of diffusing into the platelets and is associated there with intracellular proteins. Oxine and tropolone are the most common ligands used in platelet labelling, reducing neither platelet viability nor normal aggregation. Due to a strong tendency of oxine to bind to plasma components, the labelling procedure must be performed in a plasma-free medium, and the platelets must be washed in a buffer solution; by contrast, labelling of the platelets in a plasma medium is possible with tropolone. The latter method may be the safer procedure, as the necessarily repeated washing in the buffer solution during the oxine-labelling procedure may alter the platelets. A comparison of viabilities and platelet life span in In-oxine and In-tropolone labelled platelets, however, has shown no difference between the two platelet populations [48].

Labelling Procedure and Image Processing

In our laboratories we use a modified platelet-labelling procedure with ^{111}In oxine, as initially described by Thakur et al. [47] (Table 1). A quantity of 43 ml venous blood is anticoagulated with an acid citrate dextrose (formula A) solution (ACD A); platelet-rich plasma is obtained by centrifugation (180 *g* for 15 min). In a second centrifugation (900 *g* for 7 min) we obtain a compact platelet pellet which is washed in an ACD A, normal saline buffer solution (pH 6.5). The washed platelets are resuspended in the buffer solution and incubated with 500 μCi of a commercially available (Amersham Buchler, Braunschweig, FRG) ^{111}In-oxine solution (20 min at 22 °C). The labelled platelets are again centrifuged (900 *g* for 7 min) to remove the unbound radioactivity and are washed a second time in

Table 1. Method of labelling platelets with Indium 111

I. Platelet separation
1. Draw 43 ml whole blood in 7 ml ACD A solution.
2. Centrifuge, 180 *g* for 15 min.
3. Remove platelet-rich plasma (PRP) and centrifuge this, 900 *g* for 7 min.
4. Remove plasma and retain.
5. Resuspend the platelet pellet in 4 ml washing solution (3 ml ACD A + 21 ml normal saline, pH 6.5).
6. Centrifuge the washed platelets, 900 *g* for 7 min, discard supernatant.
II. Platelet labelling
1. Add 500 μCi ^{111}In-oxine (Amersham Buchler) to 5 ml washing solution and resuspend the washed platelet pellet.
2. Incubate, 22 °C for 20 min.
3. Centrifuge, 900 *g* for 7 min.
4. Remove the supernatant.
5. Resuspend the labelled platelets in plasma retained from initial separation (platelet separation step 4).
6. Centrifuge, 900 *g* for 7 min.
7. Remove plasma and resuspend the platelets in a second portion of plasma retained of the initial separation in a 5 ml syringe for injection.

autologous plasma. Finally, the labelled platelets are resuspended in the patient's plasma and reinjected intravenously.

For an estimation of platelet deposition in the carotid arteries, gamma-camera images of the neck region are recorded in an anterior-posterior projection with a conventional gamma-camera system 1 h and 24 h after the injection of the radiolabelled platelets.

Dual Isotope Technique

Due to the complex anatomical structures of the neck arteries the scintigraphic images can be misleading. As shown in Fig. 1 it is the circulating platelet-bound radioactivity which may cause false-positive as well as false-negative results. False-positive results may be caused by local vessel dilation and coiling or by crossing vessels, and false-negative results may emerge in the case of small mural thrombi overshadowed by the circulating platelet-bound activity. In order to avoid such confusing results, Peters et al. [35] have recommended the use of a dual radiotracer technique consisting of simultaneous injections of ^{111}In-labelled platelets and ^{99m}Tc-labelled red blood cells. The different energy spectra of these isotopes (^{111}In 173 keV and 247 keV; ^{99m}Tc 140 keV), enable the recording of separate gamma-camera images for both types of cells if only the higher-energy (247 keV) photons of ^{111}In are measured. The erythrocyte image represents the geometrical extent of the circulating blood pool and is identical to the platelet image, unless there is an additional thrombus-bound ^{111}In activity.

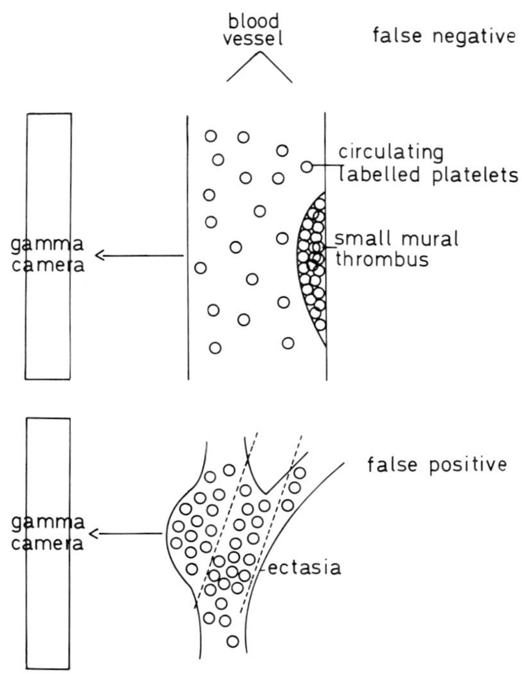

Fig. 1. Illustration of possible false-positive and false-negative results of the single-isotope technique. A false-negative result can be obtained in the case of a small mural thrombus which is overshadowed by circulating radiolabelled platelets, and a false-positive result in the case of vessel ectasia or the overlapping of two blood vessels which might imitate an accumulation of radioactivity due to thrombus formation

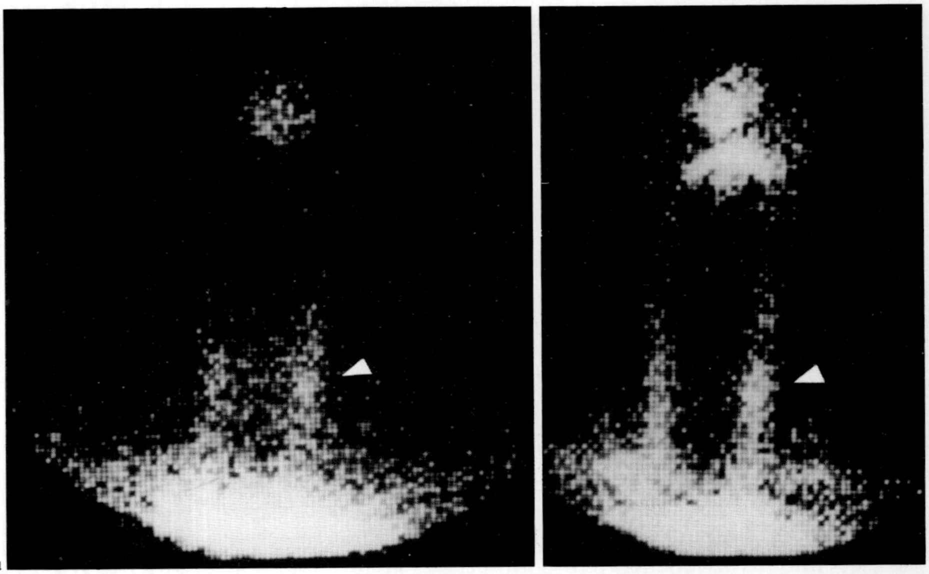

a b

Fig. 2a, b. Comparison of the ^{111}In platelet pool and the ^{99m}Tc red blood cell pool in a normal case. **a** The ^{111}In distribution in the platelet image is not exactly symmetrical: there is an increase of activity in the left carotid artery (*arrowhead*). **b** In the ^{99m}Tc blood pool image, the same increase of radioactivity can be observed on the left side (*arrowhead*). Thus, no thrombus formation can be diagnosed. At the top of both images, the nasopharyngeal blood pool, and at the bottom the aortic arch can be outlined

Figure 2a shows an ^{111}In platelet scintigram: at the bottom, the increased radioactivity of the aortic arch suggests a high number of circulating radiolabelled platelets. The image was recorded 24 h after injection of the radioactive substance. Both the major vascular neck structures and the nasopharyngeal blood pool are visible. The neck vessels are not outlined symmetrically by the radiolabelled platelets. The arrow indicates a focal increase in the left carotid artery which may represent a thrombus formation. The ^{99m}Tc erythrocyte scan, however, shows an increase in blood-pool radioactivity in this area (Fig. 2b). Thus, even the visual comparison of images indicates that there is no evidence of a pathological thrombus formation in this patient. According to Powers et al. [37], this dual isotope technique also enables quantification of platelet excess in the event of a thrombus. The measured radioactivity of ^{111}In in a region of interest (In-ROI) is equal to the sum of circulating blood-pool activity (In-BP) and the radioactivity of platelets bound to a thrombus or the vessel wall (In-EXC):

$$\text{In-ROI} = \text{In-BP} + \text{In-EXC}$$

The amount of In-BP can easily be measured by using a different radiotracer, such as ^{99m}Tc-labelled red blood cells representing the circulating blood-pool activity (Tc-BP). Since the red blood cells do not leave the circulating pool, Tc-BP is identical to the entire radioactivity measured in all regions of interest (Tc-ROI):

$$\text{Tc-BP} = \text{Tc-ROI}$$

In all reference regions (REF) not suspected of a thrombotic process (e.g., the aortic arch or the right ventricle), the ratio of isotopes, In-REF and Tc-REF, represents their relative radioactivity. The value is characterized by the amount of injected radioactive substance and the physical properties of both isotopes. Thus, in every region of interest the radioactivity due to the circulating ^{111}In platelet pool can be calculated as follows:

$$\text{In-BP} = \frac{\text{In-REF}}{\text{Tc-REF}} \times \text{Tc-ROI}$$

The excess of non-circulating, thrombus-bound ^{111}In radioactivity is then given by the following equation:

$$\text{In-EXC} = \text{In-ROI} - \frac{\text{In-REF}}{\text{Tc-REF}} \times \text{Tc-ROI}$$

A quantification of platelet excess in any region of interest is then possible. This can be important in studies monitoring antiplatelet drug effects on the thrombotic site or in cases with an uncertain visual findings. Computerized systems also allow the subtraction of the circulating blood pool from the total amount of ^{111}In radioactivity, thus making the thrombus formation visible.

Figure 3a shows a distinct accumulation of platelet-bound radioactivity in the right carotid artery (arrow) of a 50-year-old man who had experienced two right-hemispheric strokes within 2 days. In accordance with his severe left-sided hemiparesis, cranial computed tomography showed an extended hypodense area in the region of the right middle cerebral artery. Angiography showed a normal internal

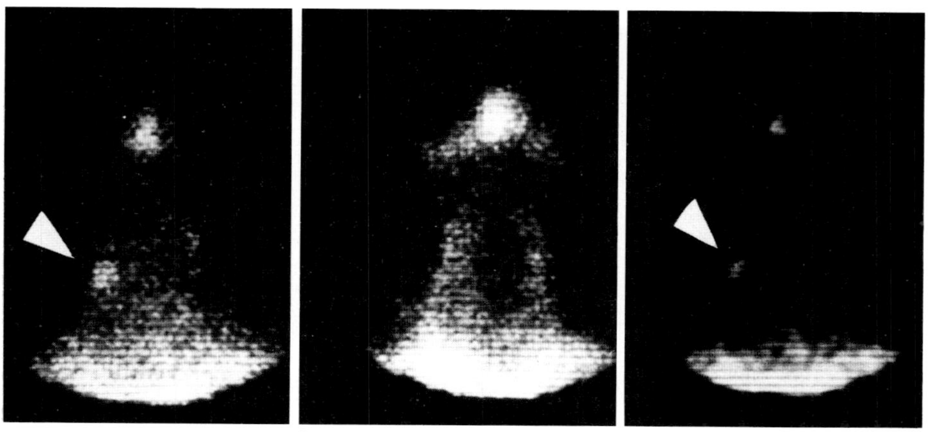

a b c

Fig. 3a–c. Pathological platelet scintigraphy in a 50-year-old man with two right-hemispheric strokes. **a** Platelet image shows a distinct platelet accumulation in the area of the right carotid artery (*arrowhead*); **b** ^{99m}Tc image demonstrates a symmetrical perfusion of both carotid arteries. **c** After subtraction of the circulating blood pool, the pure thrombus formation can be visualized (*arrowhead*) carotid artery (ICA) on the left, while a narrow plaque could be seen at the carotid bifurcation on the right with a flotating thrombus reaching into the ICA lumen. This finding could be confirmed during surgery. Figure 3 b shows the ^{99m}Tc red blood cell image with nearly symmetrical perfusion of both carotid arteries. After subtraction of the circulating blood pool the isolated thrombus formation could be visualized in the ^{111}In image.

Cardiac Images

In patients clinically diagnosed as having cardiac embolism, additional images of the heart region were performed 24, 48 and 72 h after the administration of radioactivity in an anterior-posterior and a 45° left anterior projection. In the earlier images the circulating radioactivity may overshadow a cardiac thrombus; after 48 or 72 h, however, the circulating platelet pool decreases due to withdrawal in the spleen, whereas the thrombus-bound activity increases as the thrombus continues to accumulate circulating platelets.

Figure 4 shows the cardiac platelet scintigraphy in a 65-year-old man who experienced myocardial infarctions at the age of 49 and 52 years. He was admitted to hospital after he had developed recurrent right-hemispheric as well as left-hemispheric TIA with mainly reversible neurologic deficits. Cranial computed tomography revealed hypodense areas in the territories of both middle cerebral

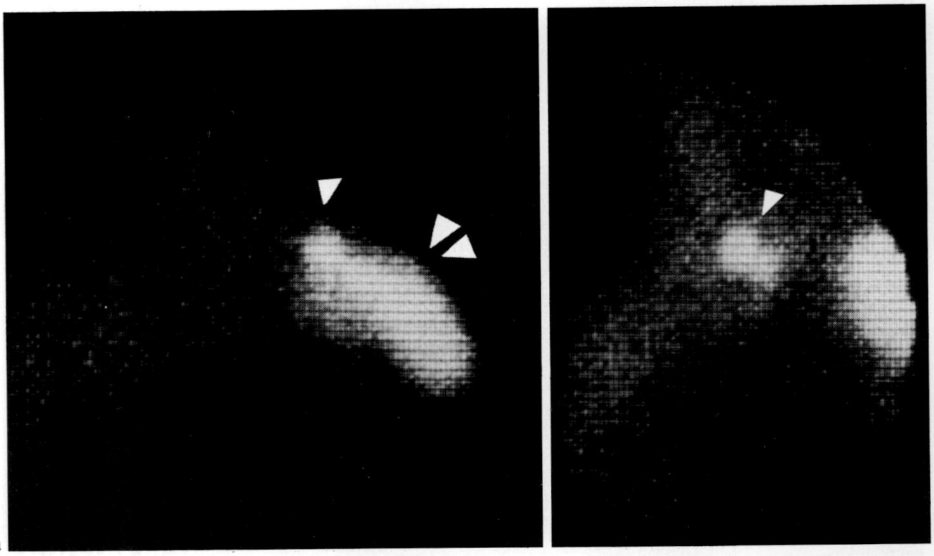

a b

Fig. 4a, b. Cardiac platelet scintigraphy in a 65-year-old patient with recurrent TIA and normal angiogram.
a Anterior-posterior projection; the left ventricular thrombus (*arrowhead*) cannot be clearly distinguished from the platelet-loaded spleen (*double arrowhead*). The liver can also be identified on the left side of the image. **b** 45° left anterior projection; the cardiac thrombus (*arrow*) can be isolated from the spleen activity. Both images recorded 48 h after injection of radiolabelled platelets

arteries; angiography of the neck vessels was normal. Two-dimensional echocardiography, however, showed a decreased ventricular contractility with thickening of the myocardium. On the 24-h scan, the anterior-posterior projection of platelet scintigraphy demonstrated an activity accumulation (arrow) near the spleen which can be seen on the right side of the image (double arrow). The increased radioactivity due to the blood pool of the liver is shown on the left. The suspected thrombus-bound platelet accumulation cannot be clearly differentiated from splenic activity. In the 45° left anterior projection, however, the thrombus can quite easily be distinguished from the activity of the platelet-loaded spleen.

Another major problem is the visualization of atrial thrombi or thrombotic deposits on the mitral valve. The small amount of platelets incorporated by the thrombi necessitate a prolongation in scanning time. Taking into account a mean platelet half-life of 8–10 days and an ^{111}In half-life of 68 h, the optimal time window to record late platelet scans seems to be 96 h after injection. During the course of these 96 h, it is possible to compare the radioactivity in the atrial space to the left ventricular radioactivity. In the case of an atrial thrombus, the atrial activity increases while the ventricular activity decreases. Figure 5 shows the cardiac platelet scintigraphy of a 48-year-old man who developed severe left-sided hemiparesis after having atrial fibrillation documented on several occasions. Angiography of brain-supplying vessels was normal. The platelet scan revealed a distinct platelet accumulation in the atrial space (arrow) showing an increase over time up to 96 h.

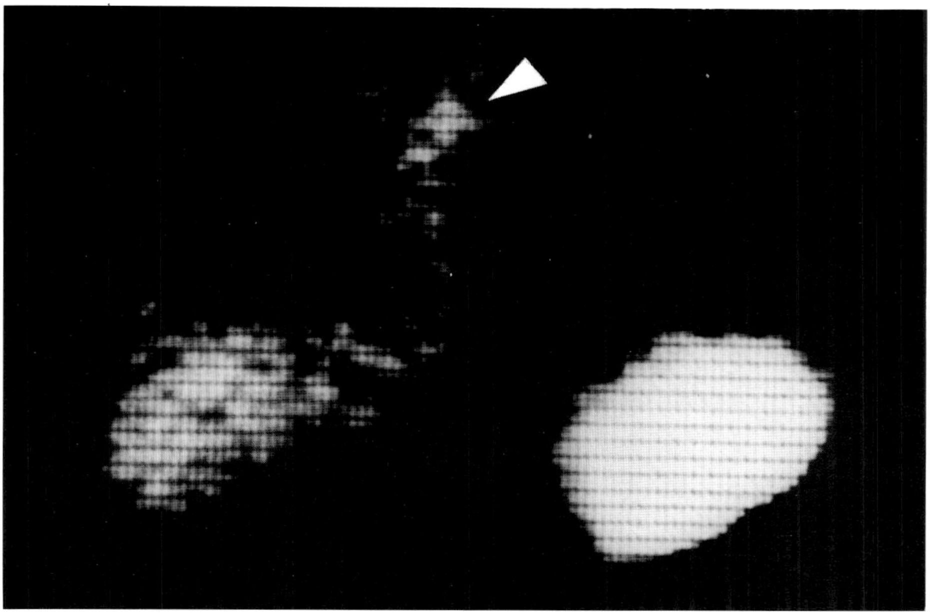

Fig. 5. Cardiac platelet scintigraphy in a 48-year-old patient with atrial fibrillation. Increased platelet-bound activity in the atrial space (*arrowhead*)

Radiation Dosage

Several authors have maintained that the total body radiation after injection of 500 µCi ^{111}In labelled platelets is negligible. The spleen, nevertheless, is the organ with the highest radiation exposure, because it is the site where platelets are stored and destroyed [31, 34]. We have evaluated the radiation exposure of different organs after injection of 500 µCi radiolabelled platelets in five patients as described by Loewinger et al. [32]. Measurements were carried out using a calculation of the absorbed dose for biologically distributed radionuclides. Scintigraphies of liver and spleen were carried out in order to calculate the biologically effective half-life of ^{111}In-bound cell components in each patient; the mean was 69 h in the spleen and 69 h in the liver, thus only slightly differing from the physical half-life of ^{111}In (68 h). Table 2 shows the average amounts of radiation exposure for several organs.

Table 2. Mean radiation exposure of critical organs after injection of 500 µCi ^{111}In-labelled platelets ($n = 5$)

Organ	Dosage (rads)
Whole body	0.26
Spleen	7.20
Liver	2.30
Testes	0.05
Ovaries	0.11

Clinical Applications in Neurology

In recent years, several attempts have been made at evaluating the clinical use of platelet scintigraphy in stroke patients [18, 23, 28, 36] with the aim of estimating the thrombotic activity of carotid atherosclerotic lesions and identifying cardiac thrombi in patients with suspected cardiogenic brain embolism.

Carotid Bifurcation Scanning

Randall et al. [39] induced carotid thrombi by electrical stimulation in rabbits. Afterwards, the thrombi were scintigraphically visualized with the help of ^{111}In-labelled platelets. Treatment with ASA or a thromboxane synthetase inhibitor led to a decrease in platelet uptake. Davis et al. [8] demonstrated positive platelet accumulations at ulcerated carotid lesions. There have been four comprehensive studies thus far dealing with platelet scintigraphy of the carotid arteries in stroke patients.

1. Powers et al. [36] examined 100 stroke patients and found pathologic platelet accumulations at the neck vessels in 52. In 87% of these, this radioactivity was observed at the site at which the atherosclerotic lesions had been documented by angiography.

2. Goldman et al. [18] performed platelet scintigraphy in 52 patients suffering from transient ischemic attacks and found a total of 26 pathologic platelet accumulations in 22 patients, 16 of which were on the symptomatic and 10 on the asymptomatic side. In 11 patients PSC was performed prior to carotid endarterectomy. In all surgery specimens an increase of radioactivity could be measured in the areas of ulcerated plaques.

3. In 1984 Isaka et al. [23] examined 25 stroke patients using the double-isotope technique. They calculated a platelet accumulation index (PAI) for several vessel segments and found a significantly higher PAI in carotid bifurcations with angiographic abnormalities than in normal ones.

4. In a preliminary study we evaluated 39 stroke patients (31 male, 8 female) with platelet scintigraphy and compared the results with angiographic and B-mode ultrasound findings. Of these, 34 had carotid territory symptoms, 23 suffering from transient ischemic attacks (TIA) and 11 from a completed stroke. Four patients had verebrobasilar symptoms and one showed an asymptomatic carotid stenosis. Thus a total of 78 carotid arteries were evaluated, 34 symptomatic and 44 asymptomatic. All symptomatic carotid arteries as well as 33 asymptomatic bifurcations were visualized by angiography. Interpretation of the scintigraphic images was carried out independently by double-blinded observers, not knowing the patient's history or the results of other imaging techniques. The observers interpreted the platelet image visually and compared it with the ^{99m}Tc red blood cell image in order to avoid false-positive results due to an enlargement of the blood pool. The observers disagreed in 6 of the 78 evaluated carotid bifurcation areas; in these cases calculation of the *In-EXC* helped to establish a positive or negative judgement. The conformity between visual and computerized analysis proved very high and statistically significant [29].

Table 3 shows the results of our findings. Angiography was normal in five symptomatic and 13 asymptomatic carotid arteries. In the five normal symptomatic carotid arteries, platelet scintigraphy was positive in four cases, showing a pathological platelet accumulation in the area of the carotid bifurcation. B-mode examination could verify intramural plaques and endothelial thickening in three of these four cases. Platelet scintigraphy was also positive in six of nine symptomatic internal carotid arteries having only slight atherosclerosis and in six out of nine symptomatic carotid arteries having low-grade stenosis ($<50\%$). In most of these cases, atherosclerotic lesions could also be demonstrated with the use of B-mode imaging. In 11 symptomatic internal carotid arteries with angiographically confirmed high-degree stenosis ($>50\%$), platelet scintigraphy was positive in about 50% of cases. Among asymptomatic cases it was less often positive; one positive scintigram out of five asymptomatic carotid arteries showed less than 50% stenosis, and two of nine pathological scans showed high-degree stenoses. Nearly all pathological platelet accumulations could be visualized in the area of the carotid bifurcation. For technical and anatomical reasons the B-mode examination failed to visualize the bifurcation area in eight vessels.

In conclusion, this study shows that platelet scintigraphy is more often positive in symptomatic atherosclerotic lesions than in asymptomatic carotid plaques. We also obtained pathological platelet scans in cases with normal

Table 3. Comparison of angiography, B-mode ultrasound and platelet scintigraphy in stroke patients ($n = 39$)

Angiography	Platelet scintigraphy				B-mode ultrasound					
	positive		negative		positive		negative		Not visualized	
	S	A	S	A	S	A	S	A	S	A
No angiography	0	0	0	11	0	1	0	9	0	1
Normal	4	0	1	13	3	3	2	9	0	1
Slight atherosclerosis	6	1	3	5	6	4	2	1	1	1
<50% stenosis	6	1	3	4	8	2	1	1	0	2
>50% stenosis	6	2	5	7	9	7	1	1	1	1

S, symptomatic internal carotid artery
A, asymptomatic internal carotid artery

angiograms or only slight atherosclerotic lesions. In most of these cases the existence of intramural atherosclerotic plaques could be demonstrated with the help of B-mode imaging. There was no difference between patients with TIA and those with stroke regarding to number of pathological platelet scans. Since all scans were carried out within 10 days after the stroke, we could not evaluate a time dependency of the incidence of pathological platelet accumulations.

Cardiac Platelet Scanning

Cardiac embolism is a frequent cause of stroke, with a high incidence of at least 20% [4]. Several cardiac diseases, such as atrial fibrillation, decreased ventricular contractility and valvular diseases, are associated with an increased risk of stroke. In a large number of cases, however, echocardiography fails to identify cardiac thrombi [9].

In an animal model, Riba et al. [40] demonstrated that the scintigraphic technique with radiolabelled platelets is a very safe method to detect experimentally induced cardiac thrombi. Ezekowitz et al. [15] studied 64 patients with ventricular aneurysms or mitral valve disease; in 46 of these they were able to demonstrate cardiac thrombi using platelet scintigraphy.

We have performed a study on 27 stroke patients with the clinical diagnosis of cardiac embolism [30]. The mean age was 55.6 years. Cardiological examination revealed a heart enlargement in 14 cases, atrial fibrillation in 10, myocardial infarction in 8, valvular disease in 4 and rheumatic disease in 3. In no case did angiography of the neck vessels reveal evidence of significant atherosclerosis. PSC identified a left ventricular thrombus in nine patients, whereas two-dimensional echocardiography (2d-E) was able only to achieve detection in three cases. Additionally, four atrial thrombi were visualized during PSC which remained undetected by 2d-E. Table 4 compares 2d-E and PSC findings. In 16 patients, 2d-E was normal, while PSC revealed four left ventricular thrombi and one atrial thrombus. Three patients with the PSC diagnosis of atrial thrombus showed valvular disease by 2d-E. Three left ventricular thrombi diagnosed during 2d-E could also be identified with the help of platelet scintigraphy.

Table 4. Correlation of 2d-E and PSC in patients with the clinical diagnosis of cardiac embolism ($n = 27$)

2d-E findings	PSC			
	LVT	AT	normal	total
Normal	4	1	11	16
DVC	2	–	2	4
LVT	3	–	–	3
MVD	–	2	–	2
AVD	–	1	1	2
Total	9	4	14	27

PSC, platelet scintigraphy
2d-E, two-dimensional echocardiography
LVT, left ventricular thrombus
AT, atrial thrombus
DVC, decreased ventricular contractility
MVD, mitral valvular disease
AVD, aortic valvular disease

These results show that PSC is a more successful method for diagnosing cardiac thrombi than is 2d-E. Simultaneous scanning of heart and neck is an advantage in identifying the source of embolism as lying either in the heart or in the carotid arteries.

Intracranial Sinus Thrombosis

Intracranial sinus thrombosis is difficult to diagnose clinically. Angiography may show some filling defects in the venous phase, but it may also be negative or inconclusive [3]. These diagnostic shortcomings may occasionally be overcome with the help of platelet scintigraphy [24]. In the majority of patients, however, angiographic, MRI and scintigraphic findings confirm one another, as can be demonstrated in the following case history.

A 39-year-old woman was admitted to our hospital after having experienced a series of generalized epileptic seizures. The patient was in a somnolent state; she had a homonymous hemianopsia on the left, a left-sided hemiparesis and a positive Babinski's sign on both sides. Cranial computed tomography only showed a slight brain atrophy. In the venous phase of the angiography, no filling of the sagittal sinus occurred, and multiple filling defects of the right transverse sinus became evident. Magnetic resonance imaging (MRI) showed an increased echo in the area of the sagittal sinus as well as in the area of the right transverse sinus (Fig. 6a). Platelet scintigraphy could also demonstrate an accumulation of platelet-bound activity in this area (Fig. 6b). Bridger et al. [2] confirmed our findings in an additional patient with superior sagittal sinus thrombosis. Since PSC is a non-invasive method, it can be used in cases with a suspected intracranial venous thrombosis. Additionally, PSC can provide further information regarding the natural history and the pathogenesis of this disease.

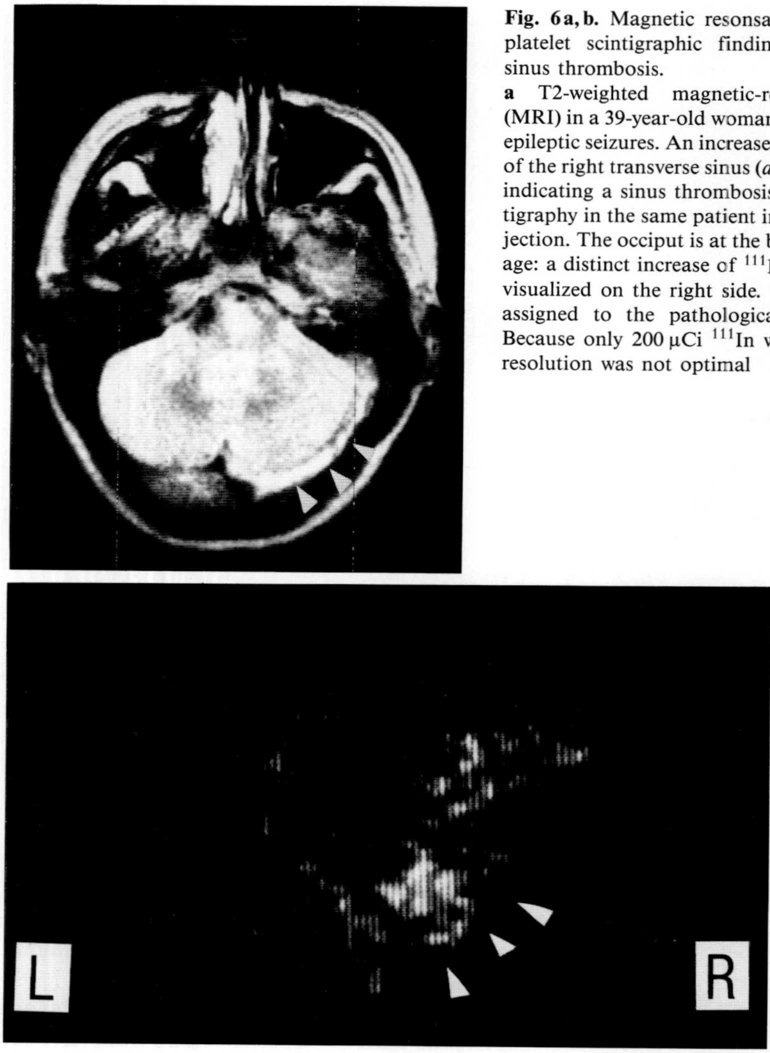

Fig. 6a, b. Magnetic resonsance imaging and platelet scintigraphic findings in transverse sinus thrombosis.
a T2-weighted magnetic-resonance image (MRI) in a 39-year-old woman with generalized epileptic seizures. An increased echo in the area of the right transverse sinus (*arrows*) is evident, indicating a sinus thrombosis. **b** Platelet scintigraphy in the same patient in a posterior projection. The occiput is at the bottom of the image: a distinct increase of ^{111}In activity can be visualized on the right side. This area can be assigned to the pathological MRI finding. Because only 200 μCi ^{111}In were injected, the resolution was not optimal

Discussion

In most stroke patients it is difficult to decide, using clinical means alone, whether cerebral ischemia has been caused by a local thrombosis or by an embolic occlusion of an intracranial artery [38]. Atherosclerotic lesions of brain-supplying arteries may serve as the source of embolism. This is also true for the heart – predominantly in the case of ventricular aneurysms, valvular disease and atrial fibrillation at the same time. As recent studies have shown, platelet scintigraphy is able to demonstrate ventricular thrombi in a high percentage of patients immediately after myocardial infarction. In many instances 2d-E fails to diagnose cardiac thrombi because these cannot be clearly distinguished from the echos of the ventricular wall [9]. This may be the reason why, in our patients, platelet scintigraphy diagnosed ventricular thrombi in 9 out of 27 cases but 2d-E in only three. Platelet scintigraphy also detected four atrial thrombi not diagnosed by preceding 2d-E. Thus our results indicate that platelet-scintigraphic scanning of the heart is an important refinement in diagnostic capability in stroke patients and helps to find cardiac, as well as extracardiac sources of cerebral embolism.

Ezekowitz et al. [14] evaluated the sensitivity of platelet scintigraphy by monitoring antiplatelet medication in patients with cardiac thrombi and found no positive effect of acetylsalicylic acid (ASA). In contrast to this finding, Cunningham et al. [6] found an ASA-induced effective inhibition of platelet deposition at sites of arterial injury after transluminal angioplasty of the iliac or femoral artery. Henningsen et al. [21] could also demonstrate decreased platelet accumulation in stroke patients treated with ASA when compared with untreated patients. These results indicate the possibility of in vivo monitoring of the effectiveness of antiplatelet drugs.

In all studies concerning carotid platelet scintigraphy in stroke patients [18, 20, 23, 27, 36] a positive correlation between scintigraphically detected platelet deposits and atherosclerotic lesions of the carotid arteries has been evident. Additionally, Goldman et al. [18] and Isaka et al. [23] also found a statistically significant correlation when the size of platelet accumulation was compared to the clinical symptoms. This remarkable finding, however, could not be confirmed by Powers et al. [36]. The reason for this discrepancy could lie in two features of the latter study: a different selection of patients, with a large number of normal angiographical findings, and an unusually long time (average, 52 days) between clinical events and scintigraphy.

In our study, the simultaneous occurrence of positive scintigrams and normal angiograms or only slight atherosclerosis in a large number of patients indicates that the clinical relevance of minor lesions may have been underestimated. The case history presented above (Fig. 3) clearly demonstrates that atherosclerotic plaques without haemodynamic relevance can promote the growth of flotating thrombi which may fragment and cause fatal cerebral infarctions. Since our patient had previously never experienced TIA, it may be wrong to state that these narrow stenoses are not capable of causing a completed stroke. In all but one of the carotid arteries having normal angiograms, or only slight atherosclerotic changes but with a positive scintigram, B-mode ultrasound examination was able to identify non-stenotic plaques. While the number of positive B-mode findings did not differ in symptomatic and asymptomatic carotid arteries, the positive platelet scans were predominantly found on the symptomatic side.

Isaka et al. [23] found the highest amount of platelet depletion in vessels with ulcerated atherosclerotic plaques, and Goldman et al. [18] could confirm these findings by means of histological examination. Animal models have shown that even small endothelial damage can cause platelet accumulations as detected by platelet scintigraphy [13]. In most cases, however, the dual radiotracer method becomes necessary in order to avoid confusing results [27].

Several methods for calculating the amount of thrombus-bound activity have been described. Sinzinger et al. [44] compared the radioactivity in a defined region of interest in both femoral arteries in patients with peripheral arterial occlusion. For carotid evaluation, however, this method does not seem to be useful due to the frequent existence of bilateral carotid atherosclerosis. Isaka and coworkers [23] calculated a "platelet accumulation index" which compares radioactivity in the region of interest with the activity in a reference region for both isotopes. In any case, this kind of analysis depends too much on the numerical fluctuation of red blood cells and does not seem to be very sensitive in measuring the platelet-bound activity. In our study we used the subtraction technique recommended by Powers et al. [37] which has the advantage of calculating platelet excess in total counts, thus enabling a comparison among various patients.

Due to the high photon-absorption of the cranial bone the detection of intracerebral thrombi using platelet scintigraphy appears difficult. In the case of sinus thrombosis, there are large thrombi, trapping a high number of radiolabelled platelets so that a thrombus visualization is made possible. Small thrombi of the cerebral arteries, however, often remain undetected. We have previously published a pathological intracerebral platelet scan of a patient with a stenosis of the middle cerebral artery [25], but such findings are very rare. Presumably, the use of single-photon computed tomography (SPECT) for the brain during PSC is a further step forward to the solution of this problem. First results in patients with peripheral arterial disease [46] seem to be encouraging.

Imaging of the vertebrobasilar system with platelet scintigraphic techniques also produces various difficulties, since most stenotic lesions in the vertebral arteries are located in their proximal part. As Fig. 2 shows, there is an overflow of radioactivity in parts of the shoulder and proximal neck region due to the aortic arch. The subclavian artery becomes evident, which hampers thrombus scanning in the initial 24 h after injection of radiolabelled platelets. Again, scanning of the neck region by a SPECT system may avoid these shortcomings.

Conclusions

PSC, as a new non-invasive imaging method, is now attracting growing interest since the imaging techniques presently in use supply information only on morphological changes, but not on the functional state of the cardiovascular system. Due to the increasing use of ultrasound technique (Doppler sonography, B-mode imaging), asymptomatic carotid artery lesions are diagnosed more frequently. As a result, the number of carotid endarterectomies also increases. Long-term follow-up studies, however, have shown that the risk to patients with asymptomatic carotid stenosis has often been overestimated.

There is a need for methods which allow differentiation between dangerous and harmless atherosclerotic carotid lesions. As several studies on stroke patients have shown, PSC of the carotid bifurcation seems to be the appropriate method for selecting high-risk patients. More detailed research is required to define the underlying morphological changes which cause platelet adherence to the lesions [20]. Another problem arises from stroke patients suffering at the same time from atherosclerosis of the neck vessels and coronary heart disease.

Simultaneous PSC scanning of both the carotid arteries and the heart may allow pinpointing the source of the embolism. A more precise diagnosis makes feasible a treatment better adapted to the pathogenesis of the stroke.

References

1. Aas KA, Gardner FH (1958) Survival of blood platelets labeled with chromium. J Clin Invest 37:1257–1268
2. Bridgers SL, Strauss E, Smith EO, Reed D, Ezekowitz MD (1986) Demonstration of superior sagittal sinus thrombosis by Indium-111-platelet-scintigraphy. Arch Neurol 43:1079–1081
3. Bousser MG, Chiras J, Bories I, Castaigne P (1985) Cerebral venous thrombosis: a review of 38 cases. Stoke 16:199–214
4. Caplan LR, Hier DB, D'Cruz JD (1983) Cerebral embolism in the Michael Reese stroke registry. Stroke 14:530–536
5. Clarke-Pearson DL, Coleman RE, Siegel R, Synan JS, Petry N (1985) Indium-111 platelet imaging for the detection of deep venous thrombosis and pulmonary embolism in patients without symptoms after surgery. Surgery 98:98–104
6. Cunnigham DA, Kumar B, Siegel BA, Gilula LA, Totty WG, Welch MJ (1984) Aspirin inhibition of platelet deposition at angioplasty sites: demonstration by platelet scintigraphy. Radiology 151:487–490
7. Danpure HJ, Osman S, Brady F (1982) The labelling of blood cells in plasma with 111-In-tropolone. Br J Radiol 55:247–249
8. Davis HH, Heaton WA, Siegel BA, Mathias CJ, Joist JH, Sherman LA, Welch MJ (1978) Scintigraphic detection of atherosclerotic lesions and venous thrombi in man by Indium-111-labelled autologous platelets. Lancet 1:1185–1187
9. DeMaria AN, Bommer W, Neumann A, Grehl T, Weinart L, Nardo S, Amstertam EA, Mason TD (1979) Left ventricular thrombi identified by cross-sectional echocardiography. Ann Intern Med 90:14–18
10. Dewanjee MK, Fuster V, Kaye MP, Josa M (1978) Imaging platelet deposition with Indium-111-labeled platelets in coronary artery bypass grafts in dogs. Mayo Clin Proc 53:327–331
11. Dewanjee MK, Rao SA, Didisheim P (1981) Indium-111-tropolone, a new high affinity platelet label. Preparation and evaluation of labeling parameters. J Nucl Med 22:981–988
12. Dewanjee MK, Solis E, Lenker J, Tidwell C, Mackey S, Didisheim P, Kaye MP (1986) Quantification of platelet and fibrinogen-fibrin deposition on components of tissue valves (Ionescu-Shiley) in calves. Trans Am Soc Artif Intern Organs 32:591–596
13. Ericus MS, Chandler WF, Ford JW, Swanson DP, Burke JC (1984) Effect of different aspirin doses on arterial thrombosis after canine carotid endarterectomy: a scanning electron microscope and Indium-111-labelled platelet study. Neurosurgery 14:198–203
14. Ezekowitz MD, Cox AC, Smith EO, Taylor FB (1981) Failure of aspirin to prevent incorporation of indium-111 platelets into cardiac thrombi in man. Lancet 2:440–443
15. Ezekowitz MD, Burrow RD, Heath PW, Streitz T, Smith EO, Parker DE (1983) Diagnostic accuracy of Indium-111-platelet scintigraphy identifying left ventricular thrombi. Am J Cardiol 51:1712–1716
16. Fitscha P, Kaliman J, Sinzinger H (1985) Gamma-camera imaging after autologous platelet labeling with 11-In-oxine sulfate: a key for assessing the efficacy of prostacyclin treatment in active atherosclerosis? In: Schrör (ed) Prostacyclins and other eicosanoids in the cardiovascular system. Karger, Basel, pp 252–357 (Proc 2nd Int Symp, Nürnberg Fürth 1984)
17. Goldman M, Hall C, Dykes J, Hawker J, McCollum CM (1983) Does 111-Indium-platelet deposition predict patency in prosthetic arterial grafts. Br J Surg 70:635–638
18. Goldman M, Leung JO, Aukland A, Hawker RJ, Drolc Z, McCollum CM (1983) 111-Indium platelet imaging, Doppler spectral analysis and angiography compared in patients with transient cerebral ischemia. Stroke 14:752–759
19. Grimley RP, Rafigi E, Hawker RJ, Drolez A (1981) Imaging of Indium-111-labeled platelets: a new method for the diagnosis of deep vein thrombosis. Br J Surg 68:714–716

20. Henningsen H, Kessler C, Reuther R, Bihl H, Allenberg J, Antalics I, Nemetschek H (1985) Indium-111-platelet-scintigraphy for detection of carotid artery atherosclerosis. In: Nestel JB (ed) Proceedings of the poster communications. 7th international symposium on atherosclerosis, Melbourne
21. Henningsen H, Kessler C, Reuther R (1986) Dual isotope scintigraphy of the carotid arteries. In: Balas P (ed) Progress in angiology. Minerva Medica, Turin, pp 95–98
22. Heyns du Pont, Loetter MG, Badenhorst PN, de Kock F, Pieters H, Herbst C, van Reenen OR, Kotze H, Minaar PC (1982) Kinetics and sites of destruction of 111-Indium-oxine-labeled platelets in idiopathic thrombocytopenic purpura: a quantitative study. Am J Hematol 12:167–171
23. Isaka Y, Kimura K, Yoneda S, Kusnucki M, Etani H, Osamu U, Tsuda Y, Abe H (1984) Platelet accumulation in carotid atherosclerosic lesions: Semiquantitative analysis with Indium-111 platelet and Technetium-99m human serum albumin. J Nucl Med 25:556–563
24. Kessler C, Kniffert T, Botch H (1980) Der Nutzen der Plättchenszintigraphie zur Aufklärung intrakranieller vaskulärer Prozesse. Akt Neurol 7:27–29
25. Kessler C, Trabant R (1982) Thrombozytensuzintgigraphyie mit Indium-111. Arch Psychiat Nervenkr 231:449–457
26. Kessler C, Reuther R, Berentelg J, Kimmig B (1983) The clinical use of platelet scintigraphy with 111-In-oxine. J Neurol 229:255–261
27. Kessler C, Reuther R, Kimmig B, Pietzsch T (1984) Dual isotope scintigraphy in stroke patients. Neuroradiology 26:113–117
28. Kessler C, Kniffert T, Reuther R, Kimmig B, zum Winkel K (1984) Die Szintigraphie mit 111-In markierten Blutplättchen. Dtsch Med Wochenschr 109:1853–1859
29. Kessler C, Henningsen H, Bihl H (1986) Interobserver reproducibility of Indium-111 platelet carotid scintigraphy and its correlation to computerized analysis. In: Reisner T, Binder H, Deisenhammer E (eds) Advances in neuroimaging. Second international congress for clinical neuroimaging Vienna. Verlag der Wiener Medizinischen Akademie, Vienna, pp 110–114
30. Kessler C, Henningsen H, Reuther R, Kimmig B (1987) Identification of cardiac thrombi in stroke patients with Indium-111 platelet scintigraphy. Stroke (in press)
31. Klonizakis J, Peters AM, Fitzpatrick ML, Kensett MJ, Lewis SM, Lavender JP (1980) Radionuclide distribution following injection of Indium-111-labelled platelets. Br J Haematol 46:595–602
32. Loewinger R, Berman M (1968) A scheme for absorbed-dose calculation for biologically-distributed radionuclides. J Nucl Med (Suppl)1:9–14
33. Panel of diagnostic application on radioisotopes in haematology, international committee for standardization in haematology (1977): recommended methods for radioisotop platelet survival studies. Blood 50:1137–1144
34. Peters AM, Klonizakis I, Lavender JP, Lewis SM (1980) Use of 111-Indium-labeled platelets to measure spleen function. Br J Haemat 46:587–589
35. Peters AM, Lavender JP (1981) Imaging vascular lesions with Indium-111-labeled platelets. Circulation 64:1297–1298
36. Powers WJ, Siegel BA, Davis HH, Mathias CJ, Clark HB, Welch MJ (1982) Indium-111-platelet scintigraphy in cerebrovascular disease. Neurology 32:938–943
37. Powers WJ, Hopkins KT, Welch MJ (1984) Validation of the dua radiotracer method for quantitative In-111 platelet scintigraphy. Thromb Res 34:135–145
38. Ramirez-Lassepas M, Cipolle RJ, Bjork RI, Kowitz J, Snyder BD, Weber JC, Stein SD (1987) Can embolic stroke be diagnosed on the basis of neurologic clinical criteria? Arch Neurol 44:87–89
39. Randell J, Wilding RJ (1980) Acute arterial thrombosis in rabbits: reducted platelet accumulation after treatment with dazoxiben hydrochloride. Br J Clin Pharmacol 15:495–499
40. Riba LA, Thakur ML, Gottschalk A, Andrile VT, Zaret BL (1979) Imaging experimental infective endocarditis with Indium-111-labeled blood cellular components. Circulation 59:336–343
41. Ritchie JL, Stratton JR, Thiele B, Hamilton GW, Warrick LN, Huang TW, Harker LA (1981) Indium-111 platelet imaging for detection of platelet deposition in abdominal aneurysms and prosthetic grafts. Am J Cardiol 47:882–889
42. Scheffel U, Tsan M, McIntryre PA (1979) Labeling of human platelets with 111-In-8-hydroxquinoline. J Nucl Med 20:524–528

43. Sinn H, Silvester DJ (1979) Simplified cell labelling with Indium-111 acetylacetone. Br J Radiol 52:758–761
44. Sinzinger H, Fitscha P (1983) Radioisotope technique for diagnosis of atherosclerosis. Giorn Arteriosclerosi 2:31–38
45. Stratton JR, Ritchie JL, Hamilton GW, Hammermeister KE, Harker LA (1981) Left ventricular thrombi: in vivo detection by Indium-111 platelet imaging and two dimensional echocardiography. Am J Cardiol 47:874–881
46. Stratton JR, Ritchie JL (1986) Reduction of indium-111 platelet deposition on Dacron vascular grafts in humans by aspirin plus dipyridamole. Circulation 73: 325–330
47. Thakur ML, Welch MJ, Joist JH, Coleman RE (1976) Indium-111-labeled platelets: studies on preparation and evaluation of in vitro and in vivo functions. Thromb Res 9:345–357
48. Vallabhajosula S, Machac J, Goldsmith SJ, Lipszyc H, Badimon L, Rand J, Fuster V (1986) Indium-111 platelet kinetics in normal human subjects: tropolone versus oxine methods. J Nucl Med 27:1669–1874
49. Webber MM, Chang D, Baffkin D, Verma A (1979) In-111-labeled platelets or iodinated fibrinogen for the detection of deep venous thrombosis. J Nucl Med 20:459–460

Platelet Scintigraphy of the Carotid Arteries: Comparison with the Histology of Thromboendarterectomy Specimens

H. HENNINGSEN [1]

Introduction

As early as 1854 Virchow described arteriosclerosis as the consequence of an abnormal interaction of circulating blood elements and the arterial wall. Although our knowledge of the pathogenesis of arteriosclerosis has since increased, it still remains to be seen what the basic mechanisms, as well as the role of platelets in the formation of atherosclerotic lesions, are. It is an accepted fact that platelets adhere and interact with subendothelial connective tissue thus promoting the formation of atherosclerotic plaques and mural thrombi [18]. The positive correlation between atherosclerotic lesions of the extracranial carotid arteries and the incidence of cerebral ischemia is well known [11]. Pathophysiologically, there are two main mechanisms thought to be responsible for causing cerebrovascular ischemia:

1. a high degree arterial stenosis resulting in a reduction of cerebral blood flow [6]
2. an "active" thrombotic or ulcerated atherosclerotic plaque which embolizes into the intracranial circulation.

Platelet emboli have been found in the retinal vessels of patients suffering from attacks of amaurosis fugax [4, 13]. However, it is often extremely difficult to define the exact etiology of cerebral ischemia in common clinical settings. Certain clinical findings can provide clues:

1. the degree of the arterial stenosis
2. the extent and surface structure of an atherosclerotic plaque
3. its composition.

Doppler sonography and angiography are well established diagnostic tools in the detection of high-degree carotid stenoses [22]. However, these two techniques cannot provide adequate biological information about atherosclerotic plaques in vivo. As of yet, B-mode ultrasound examination has not been able reliably to determine the composition of the plaques [8]. As platelets are components of atherosclerotic lesions, radiolabeling and scanning of platelets seem to be elegant methods in acquiring more information about the dynamics and composition of atherosclerotic lesions and mural thrombi. So far, some studies have given evidence of pathological platelet accumulation in about half of arteriographically abnormal internal carotid arteries [3]. Other authors have been able to show a

[1] Department of Neurology, University of Heidelberg, Voss-Str. 2, D-6900 Heidelberg, FRG

positive correlation between symptomatic internal carotid artery stenoses and pathological platelet accumulation at this anatomical site.

The clinical impact of scintigraphic platelet imaging is dependent on the causative role that platelets play in carotid artery plaque formation and secondary thrombosis. An active thrombotic process within the brain-supplying neck arteries dramatically increases the risk of brain embolism and ischemic stroke. Imparato et al. [10] examined the relationship of gross morphological characteristics and cerebral symptoms in 376 internal carotid artery plaque specimens. The only significant correlation found was the association of intramural hemorrhage with clinical symptoms. All other morphological criteria, including ulceration of the plaque, showed no significant correlation with the clinical symptomatology. This seems to contradict the findings made by Goldman et al. [5] who measured the accumulation of ^{111}In-labeled platelets in endarterectomy specimens. They found ulcerated plaques to be more active in platelet uptake than nonulcerated stenotic lesions.

In the present study, we correlated the morphological characteristics of surgically removed carotid plaques with platelet accumulation in symptomatic internal carotid arteries (ICA). The crucial question was whether platelet scintigraphy (PSC) was able to identify a certain "dangerous" type of atherosclerotic lesion which increases the patient's risk of ischemic stroke. Secondly, can we use PSC to narrow the group of symptomatic patients who would benefit from thromboendarterectomy (TEA)? In order to examine the underlying morphological changes of the vessel wall which cause platelets to adhere and accumulate, we performed light microscopy of surgical specimens obtained from 26 patients who underwent both thromboendarterectomy, as well as PSC, 1–9 days prior to the operation.

Patients and Methods

A total of 42 patients underwent thromboendarterectomy. In 26 cases a well-preserved plaque specimen was obtained during TEA. In the other 16 cases the surgical specimen could not be histologically examined because of severe mechanical impairments. Of the 26 patients whose TEA specimens were finally examined, 20 were male and 6 were female with the mean age being 56.8 years. Of these, 19 had suffered a carotid TIA and 7 a completed stroke. All patients underwent angiography of the extracranial carotid arteries.

PSC was performed 1–9 days prior to the TEA operation. In all cases the operated internal carotid artery corresponded to the symptomatic side.

The platelet-labeling procedure was established by Thakur in 1976 [20]. The modification of this method, as described by Kessler in this volume, was used in our laboratory. Scintigraphic images were recorded after the administration of radiolabeled platelets. We used a medium energy collimator which recorded at ^{111}In peaks of 173 keV and 247 keV. The procedure was performed with the patient in a supine position and anterior-posterior projection. Regions of interest (ROI) at the carotid bifurcation covered an 8×8 (i.e., 64) pixel area. The total count in each ROI was compared to the opposite side. Images were taken 1 h and

24 h after injection of the radiolabeled platelets. Each image was evaluated by two observers independently of each other, who knew neither the patient's clinical history nor the angiographic findings of the neck vessels.

The histological findings were subdivided according to the following characteristics: (a) fresh mural thrombi, (b) ulcerated plaques, (c) fibrotic plaques, (d) plaques characterized by subendothelial foam cells and extracellular lipid deposits, (e) intramural hemorrhages, and (f) mainly calcified plaques. Each characteristic was quantified as either low (+), moderate (+ +) or predominant (+ + +), using light-microscopical technique.

Results

Using PSC, 16 out of 26 examined symptomatic carotid arteries revealed a pathological platelet accumulation in the bifurcation area. The histological examination of all 26 specimens, as broken down into categories of the above-mentioned predominating characteristics, revealed four fresh mural thrombi, nine ulcerated plaques, eight fibrotic plaques, two plaques with predominant intramural hemorrhages, and three plaques with subendothelial foam cells and extracellular lipid deposits.

Table 1. Individual platelet scintigraphy (PSC) results compared to the histological findings

Patient number	PSC	Thrombus	Ulcer	Fibrous	Hemorrhage	Lipid deposit foam cells	Calcification
1	–	+ + +			+ +		
2	+	+ + +		+ +	+ +	+ + +	+
3	+	+ + +				+	+
4	+	+ + +					
5	+		+ + +		+		+
6	+		+ + +		+ +	+ +	
7	–	+	+ + +				+
8	+	+ +	+ + +				+
9	+		+ + +	+		+ +	
10	+	+ +	+ + +		+		
11	+		+ + +		+ +		+ +
12	+	+ +	+ + +				+
13	–		+ + +				+ +
14	–			+ + +			+
15	+			+ + +	+ +		+ +
16	–			+ + +		+ +	+ +
17	–			+ + +	+		+ +
18	+			+ + +	+		+
19	–			+ + +			+ +
20	–			+ + +	+ +		+ +
21	–			+ + +			
22	+	+ +	+ +		+ + +		+
23	+				+ + +		+
24	–					+ + +	
25	+	+ +				+ + +	
26	+				+ +	+ + +	+

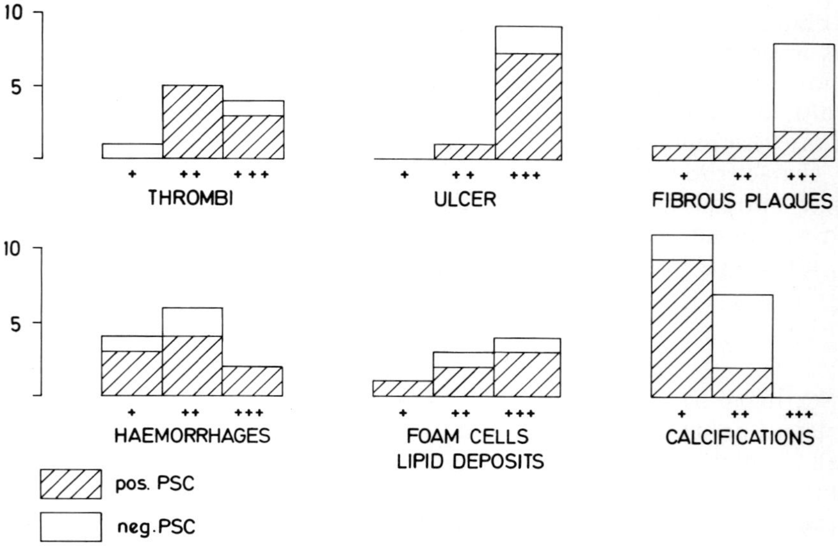

Fig. 1. Relation of cumulative PSC findings to histological criteria

Arteriography revealed only three cases with a less than 40% stenosis, six cases showed a 40%–70% stenosis, and the remaining 17 cases showed a more than 70% stenosis. The lesion, as judged by angiography, was ulcerated in five cases and not ulcerated in 21 cases. One patient, indicative of an ulcerated lesion during angiography, was shown to have a fibrotic plaque with subendothelial foam cells and calcifications (case no. 16); in the other four patients the histological findings confirmed the angiographic diagnosis.

Table 1 compares the PSC results of each patient with the histological findings. All mural thrombi (n = 10) except one large thrombus and one small thrombus (case nos. 1 and 7) showed a positive PSC. PSC was positive in three out of four cases with large mural thrombi as the predominant feature of the plaque, in seven out of nine cases with predominantly ulcerated plaques, in two out of three plaques with foam cells, and in both cases with intramural hemorrhage. However, PSC was negative in most of the predominantly fibrotic plaques (6 out of 8). Calcifications of some degree were found in nearly all plaques but predominantly in the fibrotic ones. Figure 1 shows the summary of the results.

Altogether 10 specimens revealed ulcerative lesions. Of these, two had negative and the rest positive PSCs. Out of the 13 specimens with intramural hemorrhages, 10 were positive, and only two moderate and one low-degree stenoses with intraplaque hemorrhage were negative. Plaques with subendothelial foam cells and extracellular lipid deposits more often revealed a positive PSC than a negative one.

Figure 2 shows a pathological platelet scintigram with an accumulation of radioactivity in both bifurcation areas being more pronounced on the right side than on the left. Right-side carotid thromboendarterectomy was performed in this patient. Figure 3a reveals an atheromatous plaque with an ulcer and a fibrotic

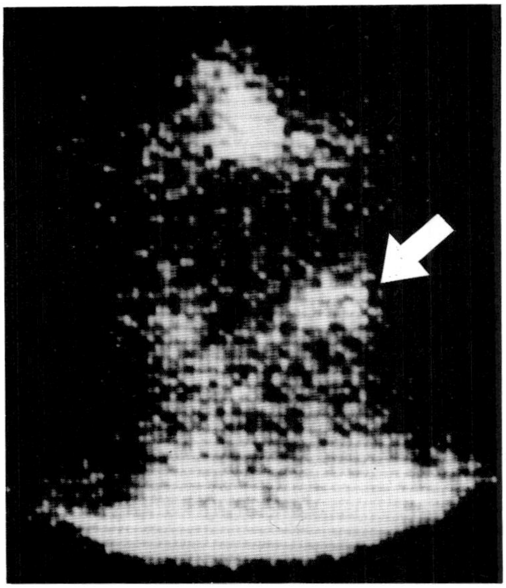

Fig. 2. Pathological platelet scintigram with an activity increase in both bifurcation areas, more on the right side than on the left

covering; in the same patient, foam cells are seen below the intima (Fig. 3b). Figure 4 shows an adhering thrombus. Conglomerates of platelets form a framework intermingled with fibrin, leucocytes and abundant erythrocytes. Figure 5 presents a typical extensive intraintimal hemorrhage (arrow), and Fig. 6 a sclerotic stable plaque in the carotid bifurcation (necropsy specimen). The same plaques are also shown in Fig. 7. These are characterized by an edematous lamina intima with extensive proliferation of connective tissue cells and hyaline transformation.

Discussion

Two out of ten histologically confirmed thrombus formations failed to be demonstrated by PSC. A further analysis of these two cases revealed either a very small thrombotic layer with ulceration or, of still more interest, a reendothelialization of the thrombus. Obviously, these morphological peculiarities of the lesions prevented sufficient accumulation of radiolabeled platelets. These findings indicate possible shortcomings with the use of PSC.

Ulcerated plaques ($n = 9$) showed a positive PSC in all but two cases. This is in accordance with the results published by Goldman et al. [5] who found a greater degree of activity of radiolabeled platelets in ulcerated plaques when compared to nonulcerated stenoses. It is difficult to interpret the significance of the negative scans in clearly ulcerated or thrombotically active lesions. In order better to explain this phenomenon we need to turn our attention to some basic methodological aspects of platelet-radiolabeling procedures:

1. With an improved scintigraphic imaging technique, Reidy et al. already obtained positive PSCs after denuding the arterial endothelial lining of an at least

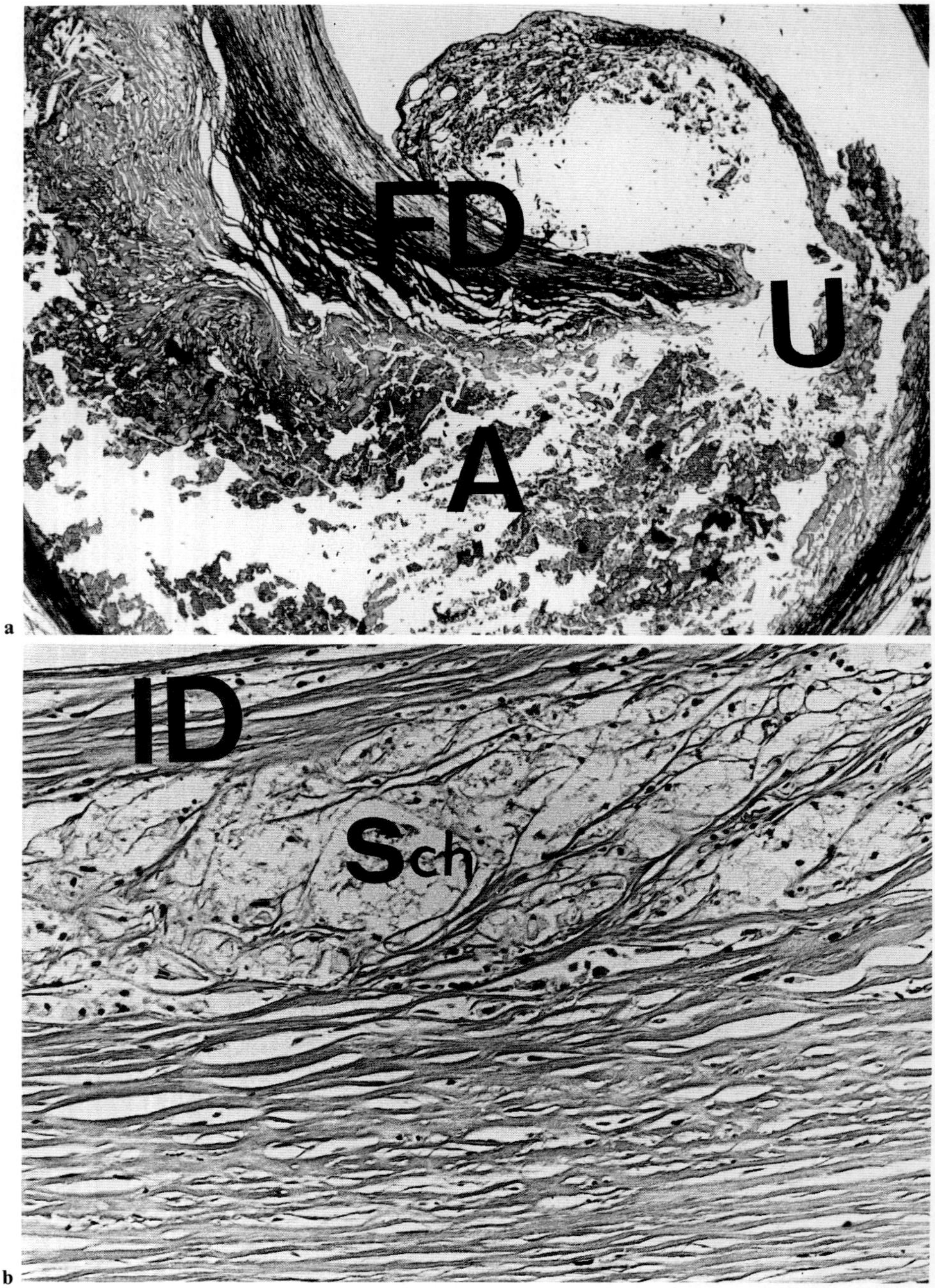

Fig. 3 a, b. Various atherosclerotic changes of an ICA plaque.
a Atheromatous plaque (*A*) with an ulcer (*U*) and a fibrotic covering (*FD*). **b** In the same patient, foam cells (*Sch*) are seen below the intima (*ID*)

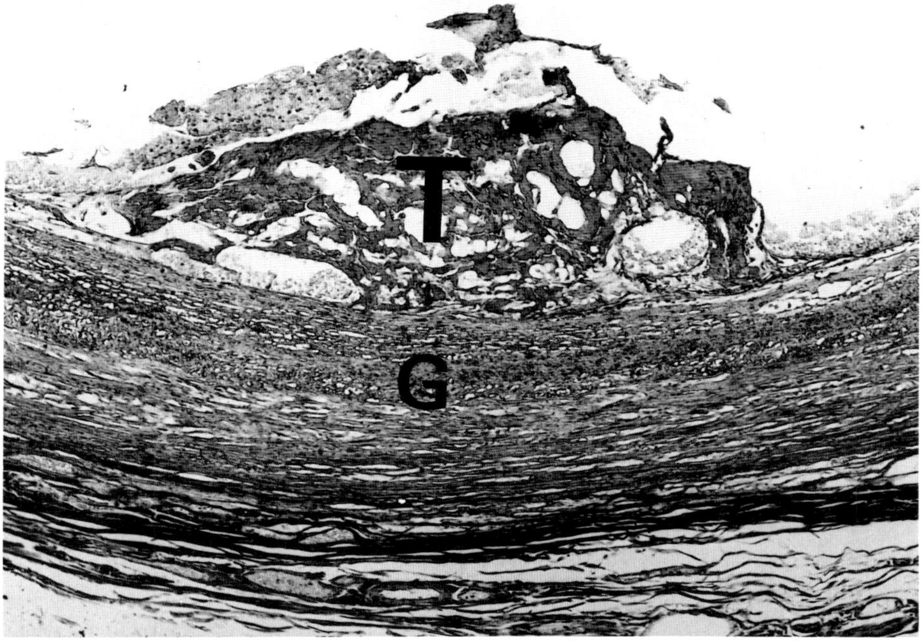

Fig. 4. Intraluminal thrombus adhering to a fibrous plaque. The thrombus (*T*) consists of conglomerates of platelets which form a framework intermingled with fibrin, leucocytes and abundant erythrocytes; *G*, vessel wall

600-cell patch [17]. Despite this increased sensitivity in PSC detection, there remains the possibility that the number of accumulated platelets was still too small to show up positively with conventional PSC in these two cases. Further animal models are required to evaluate the detection limits of various scintigraphic methods.

2. The detection of thrombi using PSC depends on the strength of focal radiolabeled platelet accumulation when compared to background noise. Thus, the sensitivity of detecting active lesions is limited by interference due to bloodborne radioactivity. In order to improve the sensitivity of PSC the circulating blood pool, as represented by ^{99m}Tc-labeled red blood cells, was subtracted to obtain the more accurate thrombus-bound activity [11, 15]. This dual radiotracer technique has already been shown to increase the accuracy of ^{111}In-platelet scintigraphy in detecting atherosclerotic lesions [9, 16].

3. An important and frequent topic of discussion in the literature refers to the efficacy of the ^{111}In-platelet labeling technique with respect to the preserved ability of the labeled platelets to adhere. During the past decade several studies have shown improvement in the labeling procedure [7, 21] which has also been recommended by the Platelet Radiolabeling Study Group [19]. Bernard, among others, has shown that the functional viability of platelets was not critically affected by new radiolabeling procedures [2].

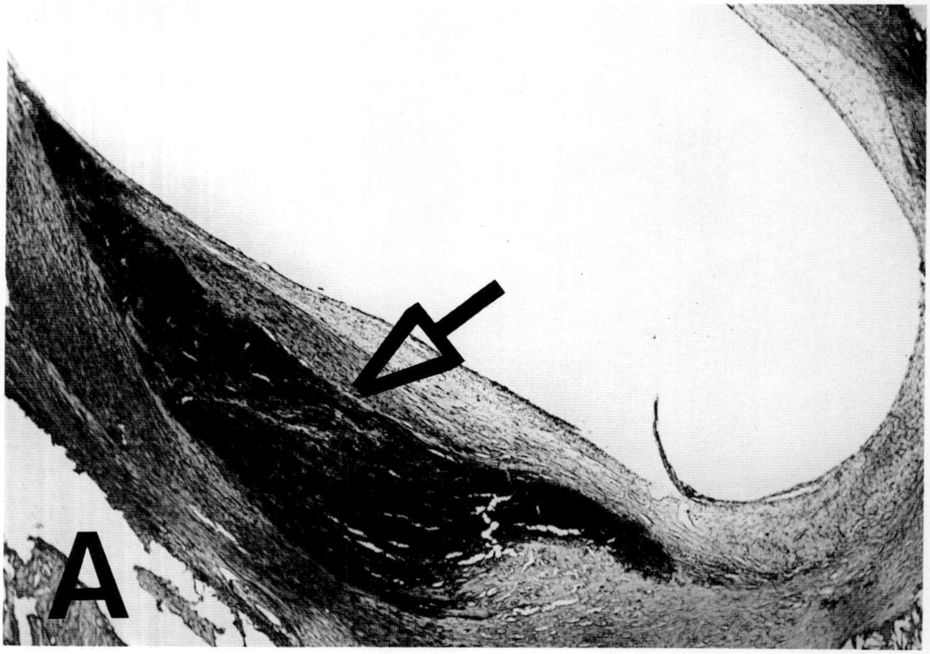

Fig. 5. Typical extensive intraintimal hemorrhage (*arrow*); *A*, atheroma

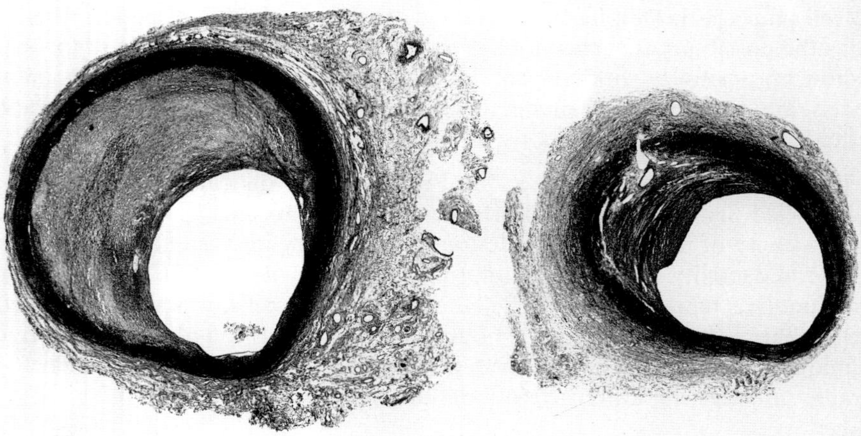

Fig. 6. Sclerotic stable plaques in the carotid bifurcation (necropsy specimen). Both the internal carotid artery (*left*) and the external carotid artery (*right*) are involved and show a moderate stenosis

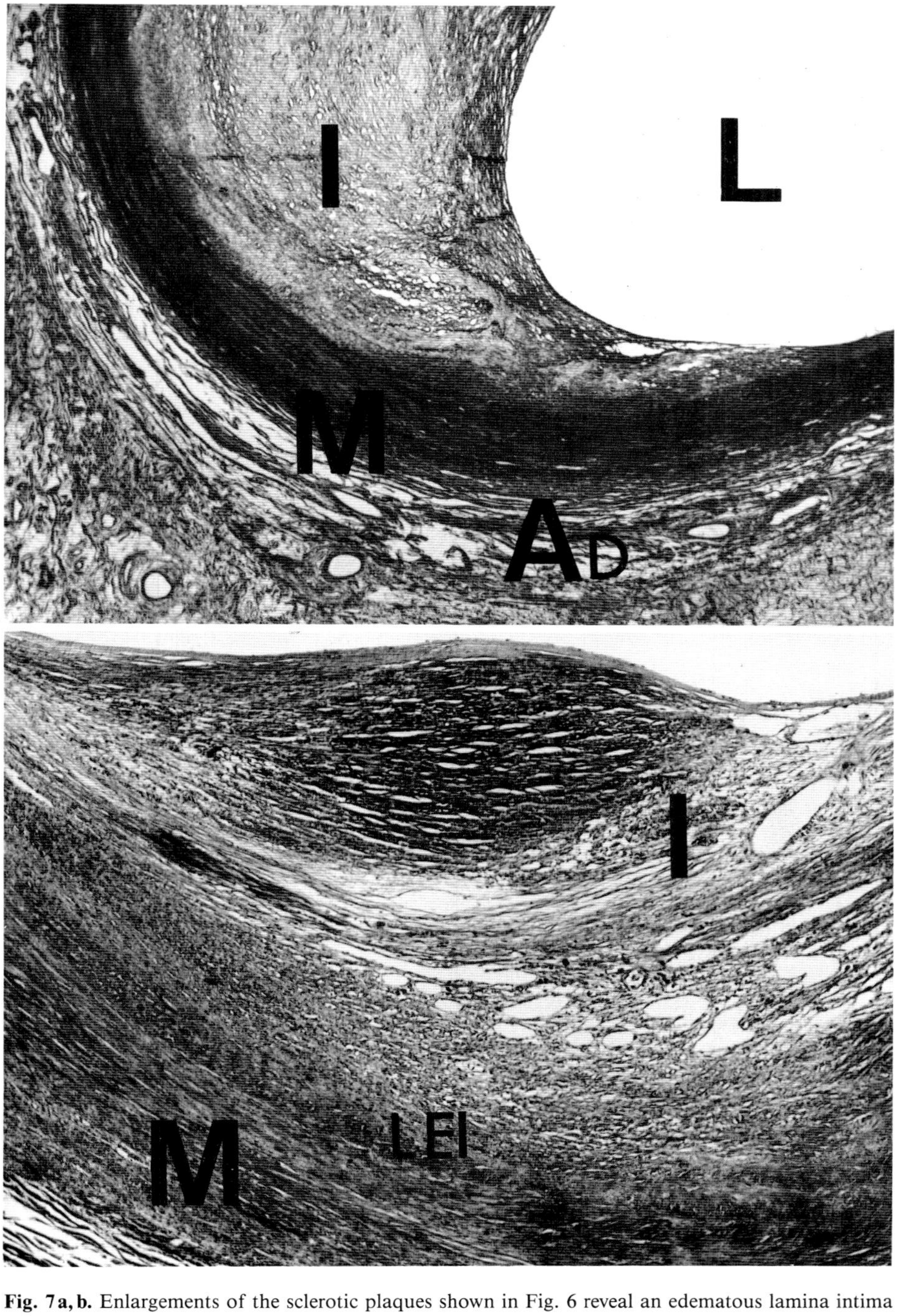

a

b

Fig. 7a, b. Enlargements of the sclerotic plaques shown in Fig. 6 reveal an edematous lamina intima with extensive proliferation of connective tissue cells and hyaline transformation. *I*, lamina intima; *M*, media; *AD*, adventitia; *LEI*, lamina elastica intima; *L*, lumen

Two predominant hemorrhagic plaques had a positive PSC. From this limited number of cases, one can only speculate that radioactive platelets may be incorporated into plaques by hemorrhages themselves, and that intramural hemorrhages are assumed to be the main factor in dramatic plaque progression [10, 14], thus inducing an acute thrombotic reaction on the plaque surface. However, the true causative relationship between hemorrhagic plaque transformation and platelet accumulation is not yet known.

Most fibrotic plaques were negative. This could indicate that PSC is able to differentiate between "active," i.e., ulcerated, and/or thrombotic plaques and "inactive" fibrotic plaques without platelet adherence. However, some PSC results seem to contradict this idea. It is possible that the negative PSC findings in some of the thrombotic lesions and ulcerative plaques are, in actuality, not false negative. This would indicate that other unknown factors also modulate platelet adherence.

Acknowledgement. I would especially like to thank Dr. I. A. Born of the Institute of Pathology, University of Heidelberg, for the preparation of expert histological slides and photographs.

References

1. Alter M, Kieffer S, Resch J, Ansari K (1972) Cerebral infarction: clinical and angiographic correlations. Neurology 22:590–602
2. Bernard P, Bazan M. Foa C et al. (1983) Functional and ultrastructural alterations of autologous platelets labeled with ^{111}In-oxine. Eur J Nucl Med 8:172–178
3. Davis HH, Siegel BA, Sherman LA et al. (1980) Scintigraphic detection of carotid atherosclerosis with Indium-111-labeled autologous platelets. Circulation 61:982–988
4. Fisher CM (1952) Observation of the fundi oculi in transient monocular blindness. Neurology 9:333–367
5. Goldman M, Leung JO, Aukland A et al. (1983) ^{111}Indium platelet imaging, Doppler spectral analysis and angiography compared in patients with transient cerebral ischemia. Stroke 14:752–756
6. Grady PA, Blaumanis OR (1983) Arterial wall changes in experimental stenosis. In: Reivich M, Urtig HI (eds) Cerebrovascular diseases. Raven Press, New York, pp 347–357
7. Hawker RJ, Hawker LM, Wilkenson AR (1980) Indium(^{111}In)-labeled human platelets: optimal method. Clin Sci 58:243–248
8. Hennerici M, Rautenberg W, Trockel U, Kladetzky RG (1985) Spontaneous progression and regression of small carotid atheroma. Lancet 1415–1419
9. Henningsen H, Kessler Ch, Reuther R (1986) Dual isotope scintigraphy (DISC) of the carotid arteries. In: Balas P (ed) Progress in angiology. Minerva Medica, Torino, pp 95–98
10. Imparato AM, Riles RS, Mintzer R, Baumann G (1983) The importance of hemorrhage in the relationship between gross morphologic characteristics and cerebral symptoms in 376 carotid artery plaques. Ann Surg 197:195–203
11. Isaka Y, Kimura K, Yoneda S et al. (1984) Platelet accumulation in carotid atherosclerotic lesions: semiquantitative analysis with Indium-111 platelets and Technetium-99m human serum albumin. J Nucl Med 25:556–563
12. Kessler C, Reuther R, Berentelg J, Kimmig B (1983) The clinical use of platelet scintigraphy with 111-In-oxine. J Neurol 229:255–261
13. Kessler C, Reuther R, Rösch M (1984) Dual isotope carotid scintigraphy in patients with amaurosis fugax attacks. Eur Arch Psychiatr Neurol Sci 234:106–111
14. Lusby RJ, Ferrell LD, Ehrenfeld WK et al. (1982) Carotid plaque hemorrhage. Arch Surg 117:1479–1487

15. Powers WJ, Mathias CJ, Welch MN et al. (1982) Scintigraphic detection of platelet deposition in atherosclerotic macaques: a new technique for investigation of antithrombotic drugs. Thromb Res 25:137–142
16. Powers WJ (1984) In-111 platelet scintigraphy: carotid atherosclerosis and stroke. J Nucl Med 25:626–628
17. Reidy MA, Yoshida K, Harker LA, Schwartz SM (1986) Vascular injury: quantification of experimental focal endothelial denudation in rats using Indium-111-labeled platelets. Arteriosclerosis 6:305–311
18. Ross R (1986) The pathogenesis of atherosclerosis: an update. N Engl J Med 314:488–500
19. Snyder EL, Moroff G, Simon T et al. (1986) Recommended methods for conducting radiolabeled platelet survival studies. Transfusion 26:37–41
20. Thakur ML, Welch MJ, Joist JH, Coleman RE (1976) Indium-111-labeled platelets: studies on preparation and evaluation of in vitro and in vivo functions. Thromb Res 9:345–357
21. Thakur ML, Walsh L, Malech HL, Gottschalk A (1981) Indium-111-labeled human platelet: improved method, efficacy and evaluation. J Nucl Med 22:381–385
22. Weaver RG, Howard G, McKinney WM et al. (1980) Comparison of Doppler ultrasonography with arteriography of the carotid bifurcation. Stroke 11:402–404

Thrombosis and Cerebrovascular Disease*

W. HACKE[1,2], G. J. DEL ZOPPO[1,2], and L. A. HARKER[1]

Introduction

Vascular endothelial-hemostatic interactions are important in maintaining uninterrupted cerebral blood flow. Alterations in the integrity of the endothelium of brain-supplying arteries may compromise flow secondary to platelet aggregation, activation of the coagulation system, or changes in the erythrocyte or leukocyte constituents of the blood with consequent thrombotic occlusion leading to cerebral ischemic tissue injury [1–3]. The majority of acute strokes are pathogenetically related to atherothrombotic or thromboembolic events [4–6]. The location and extent of the territory suffering ischemia is determined by the presence, the type and the degree of arterial collateralization [7–8]. Hemorheologic considerations may also affect the extent of cerebral tissue injury. This review outlines the role of thrombosis in acute stroke, some of the characteristics of the cerebrovascular anatomy important for the development of ischemic stroke, and the basis for the use of antithrombotic agents in the treatment of cerebral ischemia.

In general, the important flow-limiting events include atheroma formation, in situ thrombosis, and thromboembolism. Atheroma formation may produce cerebral ischemia by three mechanisms: (a) arterial stenosis with consequent impairment of blood flow, (b) embolism of atherothrombotic material, and (c) in situ thrombosis. Atheromata of the extra- and intracranial arteries have a predilection for the carotid bifurcation, the carotid siphon, specific portions on the circle of Willis, and the proximal middle cerebral artery [9, 10]. The hypotheses of atherogenesis have been reviewed elsewhere [11].

Both thrombus formation and arterial stenosis (as the basis for hemodynamically induced cerebral lesions) imply underlying vascular endothelial damage [9, 11, 12]. Endothelial denudation may occur secondary to mechanical (including shear stress), immunological, chemical, or infectious processes. Endothelial injury leading to local thrombosis may be caused by specific antibodies, circulating

* This work was supported in part by the Deutsche Forschungsgemeinschaft grant No. Ha 1394/2-1 (W. Hacke) and grant No. Aa-2/75-1 (G. J. Del Zoppo), and by the NIH grant No. HL31950 and RR00833.
* This is publication number 4696BCR from the Research Institute of Scripps Clinic, La Jolla, California.

[1] Department of Basic and Clinical Research, Scripps Clinic and Research Foundation, 10666 North Torrey Pines Road, La Jolla, CA 92037, USA
[2] Department of Neurology, Klinikum RWTH, D-5100 Aachen, FRG

immune complexes (e. g., arteritides), or sensitized lymphocytes as well as by conditions such as hyperlipidemia, homocysteinemia, or hypoxemia [13, 14]. Bacteria and viruses either directly or by means of endotoxins or immunological reactions may also induce activation of the coagulation system [15].

Thromboembolism, another contributor to cerebral ischemia, arises from atherothrombotic fragments of proximal arterial atheromatous plaques or from cardiac mural thrombi. Thromboemboli from the large extracranial arteries to the intracerebral arteries, such as the middle cerebral artery, may be secondary to in situ thrombolysis. Thus the relative importance of the processes of thrombosis, thrombolysis, and thromboembolism in the cerebral vasculature are determined by the presence of local vascular disease, hemodynamic factors, the presence of arterial collaterals, and the vascular and systemic activation mechanisms affecting platelets, coagulation, and fibrinolysis.

Mechanisms of Thrombosis and Thromboembolism

Thrombus growth is dependent upon the dynamic balance between thrombus formation and thrombus dissolution [1–3, 16, 17] (Fig. 1). Generally, thrombus formation (e.g., in situ thrombosis) requires activation of both platelets and coagulation factors [18–20] while thrombus size is limited by the processes of embolization and thrombolysis. Embolization results from intrinsic fibrinolysis and shear forces in the microenvironment of the thrombus to produce downstream translocation of thrombus fragments [21]. Once a thromboembolus has lodged, the processes of thrombus growth and dissolution continue at the new site.

Platelet Adhesion and Aggregation

Exposure of subendothelial collagen and connecting tissue secondary to endothelial injury stimulate local platelet adherence, release, and aggregation [22, 23]. Platelet activation involves a conformational change in the platelet-membrane glycoprotein complex GPIIb/IIIa thereby exposing the fibrinogen receptor which mediates platelet aggregation [27, 28]. It also results in the release of dense granule ADP and α-granule constituents (e.g., platelet factor 4, PDGF, β thromboglobulin) and the activation of a platelet-membrane phospholipase complex which generates thromboxane A_2 [24–26]. Circulating platelets are recruited to the growing platelet thrombus through the synergistic action of released ADP, thromboxane A_2, and thrombin formed on adherent activated platelets (see below). The growing platelet thrombus is stabilized by the effects of thrombin on fibrinogen to form fibrin, and its stabilization by platelet-associated factor XIII. Other adhesive proteins that may be associated with platelet interactions include fibronectin, von Willebrand factor, and thrombospondin [28, 29].

Coagulation System Activation

Thrombin plays a central role in thrombus formation. Thrombin is generated locally on the platelet surface through both extrinsic and intrinsic pathways of coagulation. All injured cells release tissue thromboplastin to activate extrinsic coagulation; Hageman factor is activated both by disrupted endothelial cells and by subendothelial connective tissue to initiate intrinsic coagulation [30]. Platelets promote subsequent activation of the early stages of intrinsic coagulation by a process that involves a factor XI receptor and high-molecular-weight kininogen. Platelets provide a phospholipid surface which binds specifically factors V and VIII and facilitate the activation of factor X to Xa. Low concentrations of thrombin, sufficient to stimulate platelet release of α-granules but not cleave fibrinogen, are formed on the platelet surface within seconds of exposure to non-endothelialized surfaces. Thrombin-modified factor V (factor Va) is platelet-bound and serves as a high-affinity platelet receptor for factor Xa, which together with factor Va mediates a 10^5-fold increase in thrombin generation [31–34]. Thrombin-mediated cleavage of fibrinogen results in fibrin formation and thrombus stabilization.

Other local mechanisms in association with endothelial cell and tissue injury may release tissue thromboplastin and activate the extrinsic coagulation system thereby contributing to thrombin formation. Traces of thrombin produce activation of factors V and VIII on the platelet surface to accelerate thrombin generation by positive feedback pathways. Additional amplification may result from tissue factor activation of factor VII, and, subsequently, of factors IX and X. It is apparent that thrombin generation and, therefore, thrombus formation result from a number of simultaneously and variously interacting molecular mechanisms [33].

Intrinsic Thrombolysis

Limitation of thrombus growth and thrombus dissolution result from the activation of fibrin-coupled plasminogen within the thrombus [35]. Both fibrin and platelet-bound plasminogen are activated by fibrin-bound tissue plasminogen activator (tPA) and the local effect of single-chain urokinase plasminogen activator (scuPA) [36–38]. Plasmin, a serine protease, mediates fibrin degradation with the formation of oligopeptide fragments of fibrin cleavage. Modulation of thrombus-limited thrombolysis occurs by the inhibition of plasminogen activators by a family of inhibitors, of which several (platelet derived and nonplatelet derived) have been isolated [39]. Conversely, an increase in tissue plasminogen activator activity from human endothelial cells is mediated by thrombin and relative reduction of the activator inhibitor activity [40]. Finally, circulating plasmin is inactivated by α_2-antiplasmin and nonspecifically by α_2-macroglobulin, which serve to limit thrombolysis to the fibrin-containing thrombus [38]. Therefore, thrombus dissolution results from the local release and stimulation of plasmin within the thrombus where it is protected from inactivation by circulating inhibitors.

Limitation of Thrombus Growth

In addition to the mechanisms of thrombolysis noted above, limitation of thrombus growth and of distally embolized thrombi occurs by a number of mechanisms: (a) inactivation of thrombin by circulating plasma protease inhibitors, (b)

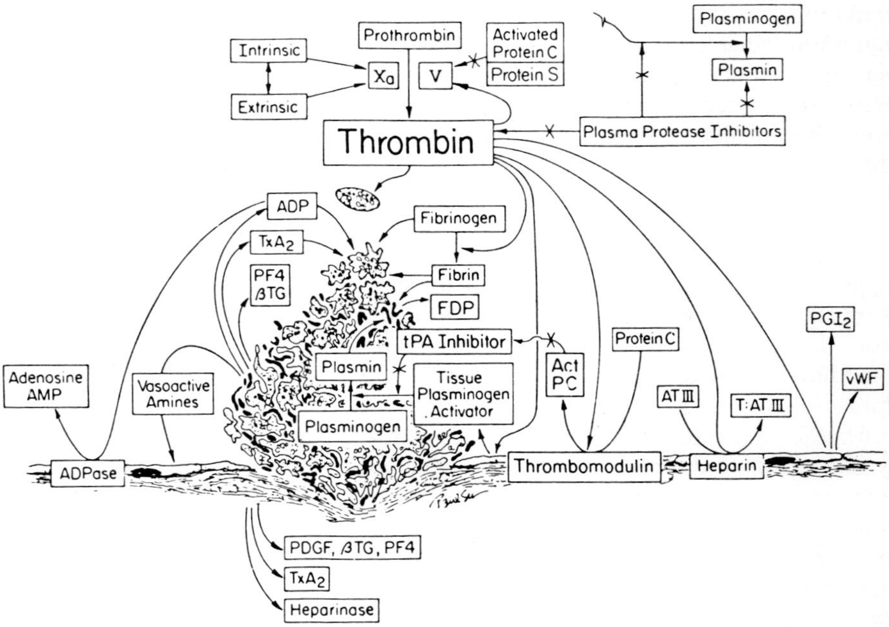

Fig. 1. *Mechanisms limiting thrombus extension.* Intact endothelium actively resists thrombus formation. Platelet aggregate formation is prevented by the endothelium despite the presence of ADP, epinephrine or thrombin through the inactivation of ADP, active clearance of vasoactive amines, facilitated complexing of thrombin with antithrombin III and the explosive thrombin-mediated synthesis and release of inhibitory PGI_2. These mechanisms markedly decrease the possibility of thrombus forming in the presence of intact endothelium. The potent effects of thrombin are also actively limited to the site of vascular injury by plasma protease inhibitors, enhancement of the endothelial surface of thrombin-antithrombin III complex formation, binding of circulating thrombin to thrombomodulin (a receptor of luminal surface of the endothelial cells) thereby activating protein C to destroy factors V and VIII and induced release of tissue plasminogen activator from vascular endothelium. Thus, thrombin initiates negative feedback mechanisms controlling its own generation. (From [102])

inactivation of plasma and platelet-bound factors Va/VIIIa by activated protein C, and (c) thrombin-antithrombin III complex formation, mediated at the adjacent endothelial surface [38, 41, 42]. APC is generated by the action of thrombin on protein C via the endothelial receptor, thrombomodulin [40]. Protein S is an important cofactor for activated protein C. In addition, the intact endothelium acts as a barrier to thrombus growth through inactivation of the platelet proaggregant ADP (with generation of adenosine and AMP), removal of platelet-dependent vasoactive amines, and the production of the platelet aggregation antagonist prostacyclin (PGI_2) [43]. Hereditary deficiencies of substances participating in the processes of thrombolysis or of thrombus growth limitation such as protein C deficiency, protein S deficiency, and antithrombin III deficiency correlate with a strong tendency toward thrombotic cerebral arterial ischemic events or recurrent cerebral venous sinus thrombosis [41]. Furthermore, the incorporation of fibrin(ogen) breakdown fragments into forming thrombus, leads to a necessarily destabilized thrombus, thereby limiting its extension. While these processes contribute significantly to the limitation of thrombus extension, and may contribute to thrombus destabilization and fragmentation, they are insufficient by themselves, as they require adequate blood flow to remove inhibitor complexes and thrombus fragments thus formed. The converse condition (stasis of flow) leads to thrombus formation, growth, and extension.

Hemorheology and Arterial Thrombosis

The primary role of hemorheologic disturbances in thrombus formation is best illustrated by the effect of stasis on thrombus growth. Furthermore, the development and localization of thrombi may be influenced by the hemodynamic stresses on vessels. Disturbed blood flow patterns at the site of irregularities in the vessel wall, or at stenoses or bifurcations have been extensively studied [44]. The flow pattern of blood may contribute to the formation and localization of atheromata and thrombi by producing: (a) areas of low flow or stasis, (b) possible damage to the formed components of blood at areas of very high flow and shear stress, and (c) damage to the vessel wall [44]. While it is unclear whether atherogenesis occurs preferentially at sites of high or low shear stress [45], it is apparent that bot the macroscopic and the microscopic appearance of a thrombus depends on the velocity of the blood stream in which it is formed [46]. Very high shear stresses and flow rates occur at the edge of obstructions and may cause erythrocyte deformation and damage, and possibly platelet activation and endothelial damage [47, 48]. The relationship of hemorheological factors to *arterial* thrombosis is complex and not fully known. An elevated whole-blood viscosity caused by either high hematocrit, even within the so-called normal range, or a high plasma fibrinogen is an important risk factor in arterial thrombosis in the cerebral vasculature [44, 46].

Hemodynamic stresses may act on the formed elements to trigger thrombogenesis [49]. Shear stress may damage and activate platelets (shear damage) thereby causing release reaction and aggregation before there is any irreversible damage to normal red cells [47]. Activated and unactivated platelets are transported toward the vessel wall along radially oriented streamlines, ultimately reaching a stagnation point at which platelet adhesion occurs. Platelet accumulation is enhanced in conditions of an increased hematocrit [50], which in regions with high shear rates platelet deposition is decreased. The general transportation rate of platelets to this point is not diminished, rather physical removal of platelets from the surface ("tearing them off") or inadequate residence time limit deposition [45, 50]. Platelet aggregation and thrombosis may also be initiated by ADP released from damaged erythrocytes. This might occur at the orifice of atheromatous stenoses or at sites of hemorrhage in atheromatous plaques where hemodynamic stresses may cause the release of erythrocyte ADP from cells undergoing extreme deformation or hemolysis [51]. Platelet activation would be expected to take place in regions of high shear stress while thrombus formation should occur at the stagnation point.

Finally, hemorheological factors may play a secondary role in the extent of the region of cerebral ischemia. During acute cerebral ischemia any increase in fibrinogen leading to an increase of whole-blood viscosity may decrease perfusion of the marginally ischemic area (penumbra) around the thrombosed vascular segment and thereby determine the final extent of tissue infarction, in addition to steal effects, vasoparalysis, and acidosis.

Evidence regarding the contributions of hemorheologic factors to the specific events of cerebral arterial thrombogenesis is inconclusive. It is difficult to isolate the relevant fluid-dynamic factors of shear rate and shear stress, flow patterns and flow distributions, and the thickness of the fluid and diffusion boundary layers under clinical conditions. Which coagulation proteins are most relevant in a given flow situation, on which vascular or platelet surfaces they are activated, and the local concentration and eventual fate of secreted platelet products in a given situation, are not known [46].

Brain-Supplying Arteries and Thrombosis

While the molecular processes of thrombus formation, growth, extension, destabilization, and fragmentation are rather uniform within the arterial system, their consequences in the *cerebral* vasculature are dependent upon the unique characteristics of the cerebral arterial (pathological) anatomy.

Ischemic stroke may result from (a) atherosclerotic diseases of the large extracranial blood-supplying vessels, (b) diseases of the large intracranial vessels, (c) diseases of the small intracerebral arteries, and (d) from cardiogenic thromboemboli [5, 7, 52] (see also Ringelstein, this volume). Differences in expected sites of endothelial damage, reduced blood flow, and coagulation activation as described above, may occur in the extracranial, intracranial, and small-caliber intracerebral vessels. Also, the clinically apparent consequences of cerebral arterial thrombosis may rely upon the presence of a collateral vascular network capable of bidirectional blood flow.

The vasoarchitecture of the intracerebral arteries differs from that of the extracranial arteries. Compared to extracranial vessels of similar luminal diameter the thickness of the intracerebral arterial wall decreases significantly once the artery has reached the endocranium. The wall diameter of the intracranial vertebral artery is reduced by more than 60%, due mainly to a decrease in adventitial substance and, to a much lesser degree, to a sparing of the muscularis mucosa. In contrast, the intima and the endothelium are not apparently different from those of the extracranial arteries. Therefore, the vessel-wall constituents responsible for platelet activation steps and thrombus formation are not different among the different intracranial arteries. The muscularis mucosa, involved in atheroma formation, is less prominent in the more peripheral intracranial vessels. This may underlie the predominance of atheromatous stenoses at extracranial artery sites and in the large proximal intracranial arteries such as the basilar artery and the proximal middle cerebral artery.

Endothelial damage in the large extra- and intracranial vessels is prominent in segments in which branching or division of the vessels takes place. This is due to irregularities in the circular winding of the muscularis mucosa, which, under the influence of shear stress and hypertension, lead to dilatation, pseudoaneurysm formation, and endothelial damage [53–56]. A prominent role of smooth muscle cell growth, proliferation, and migration mediated by platelet-derived mitogens (e.g., PDGF) in some of these processes has been suggested [54].

Little is known about the differences in distribution and concentration of endothelial factors affecting thrombus formation in the microvasculature (e.g., capillaries and precapillary arterioles) where a dramatic increase of intravascular surface and reduction of blood flow velocity is responsible for a much longer exposure of a unit volume of blood to the endothelial surface. Microvascular thrombotic occlusion has, however, been demonstrated in regions of functional endarteries (e.g., the lenticulostriate arteries) of the proximal parent artery (e.g., proximal middle cerebral artery) when ischemia/infarction of the dependent territory has been produced. It remains unclear how, under physiological circumstances, thrombus formation is inhibited in the low-flow state of the microvasculature [46].

A unique aspect of the cerebral arterial blood supply is the presence of collateral arterial networks which may modulate the expected effects of cerebral arterial thrombosis:

1. The pial collateral network can establish retrograde collateral blood flow via the long circumferential arteries. Additionally, the circle of Willis provides basal collateral blood flow [57–59]. Thus, in some situations occlusion of one, two, or even three major brain-supplying intra- or extracerebral arteries can be tolerated symptom-free in the presence of a well established network of intracranial collaterals.
2. There are numerous physiological collaterals from extracranial extracerebral arteries that can be activated in cerebrovascular occlusive disease [60, 61].
3. Occlusion of small noncollateralized perforating vessels can be followed by significant clinical deficit, while the occlusion of more proximal feeding arteries does not necessarily cause an ischemic deficit depending on the state of collateralization. Therefore, reduction of thrombus size and downstream propagation of thrombus fragments which is tolerable in other organs can cause neurological manifestations or an increase in a preexisting neurological deficit due to cerebral ischemia.

Pathological conditions particularly associated with in situ cerebral arterial thrombosis provide insight into functional aspects of the vascular microanatomy. Vessel wall changes of the small perforant arteries found in hypertension are qualitatively different from atherosclerosis of the larger vessels. The endothelium in the cerebral vascular tree is not uniform. The interendothelial spaces in small arteries and arterioles, but not in capillaries, provide a route for passage of substances that may be enhanced in hypertension [62]. During short-term hypertensive periods extravasation of serine proteases and erythrocytes secondary to endothelial damage or transendothelial vesicular transport is enhanced [56, 62]. During long-term hypertension the lumen of the small vessel may become occluded by the subintimal accumulation of hyalin substances ("lipohyalinosis") resulting in weakening and disintegration of the vessel wall, and, in some cases, total vascular occlusion [63, 64]. Additionally, endothelial damage can promote in situ intraluminal thrombosis.

Inflammatory states affecting the muscularis mucosa and basal membrane produce endothelial damage and exposure of subendothelial structures and may lead to in situ thrombosis. The sites of endothelial damage in this setting differ from those of atheroma formation. Multiple segmental stenoses and occlusion of distal branches of the long circumferential arteries are the most prominent findings in association with inflammatory vascular states, probably due to endothelial damage induced by toxic products of leukocytes or immunological injury [13, 14]. The thrombotic processes in giant-cell arteritis, for instance, may occur in either large extracranial or large intracranial vessels.

Finally, thromboembolic occlusions are found at sites where the intravascular lumen changes rapidly (e.g., bi- or trifurcations of large vessels, such as the carotid bifurcation, the carotid "T" or C1 segment, the middle cerebral artery trifurcation, the top of the basilar artery) or in the neighborhood of stenoses. Partial lysis of those "parent" thromboemboli, again, can lead to downstream (second-stage) embolism of thrombus fragments into smaller vessels.

Antithrombotic Therapy

A number of agents with anticoagulant, antiplatelet, or fibrinolytic activity have been used to modulate the thrombotic process in patients with cerebrovascular thrombotic disease [65]. The rationale for their use in the various manifestations of thrombotic/thromboembolic cerebrovascular disease has not always relied upon an understanding of the mechanisms of thrombus generation in a given setting.

A brief discussion of the more commonly used antithrombotic agents, their mechanisms of action, and their relationship to cerebrovascular disease follows. The evidence for specific uses listed for each agent continues to accumulate and therefore is subject to change (Table 1).

Anticoagulants

Heparin

Heparin is a family of mucopolysaccharides with a molecular weight range between 6×10^3 and 14×10^3 daltons and a plasma half-life of 30–60 min when administered intravenously [66, 69]. Its anticoagulant activity is mediated through binding to antithrombin III (AT III), thereby facilitating the inactivation of thrombin, factors VIIIa, IXa, Xa, and XIa, and plasmin [67]. Antithrombin III itself is activated in the presence of thrombin [68]. Significantly, antithrombin III deficiency can be associated with intravenous thrombosis, arterial thrombotic occlusions, or intracerebral arterial thrombosis [69]. Heparin therapy is monitored by the aPTT (activated partial thromboplastin time) [70].

Since heparin is an anticoagulant it is most commonly used in nonseptic cardiogenic thromboembolic cerebrovascular disease and cerebral sinus thrombosis [71, 72]. Heparin is also used to prevent thrombus extension at the site of preexisting arterial stenosis, such as high-grade carotid bifurcation stenosis, carotid

Table 1. Differential treatment of thrombotic-thromboembolic stroke

Condition/pathogenesis	Agents[a]				
	Antiplatelet	Anticoagulant	Fibrinolytic	Hemorheologic	Other
TIAs, TIAs associated with low-or mediumgrade carotid stenosis	X[b]				
TIAs, minor stroke[c] associated with high-grade carotid stenosis (common, bifurcation, internal), prior to endarterectomy		X			
TIAs, minor stroke, progressing stroke, all associated with intracranial stenosis such as ICA, MCA, VA, BA		X			
TIAs, stroke associated with embolic cardiac disease		X			
Acute stroke (<6h) due to thrombotic or thromboembolic occlusion of a major intracerebral artery (ICA, MCA, BA)			X		
Microangiopathies (lacunae, SAE)				X	
Hemodynamically induced TIAs and stroke associated with high grade ICA stenosis prior to endarterectomy				X	
Hemodynamically induced stroke in posterior circulation, prior to PTA and/or operation		(X)		X	
Hyperviscosity syndrome, hyperfibrinogenemia				X	
Antithrombin III, protein C deficiencies		X			AT III
Vasculitis				X	Immunosupp.

[a] Agents (most commonly used agents in italies):
Antiplatelet agents: *ASA*, *dipyridamole*, sulfinpyrazone, ticlopidine; Anticoagulants: *heparin*, *coumarins*; Fibrinolytic agents: *streptokinase, urokinase,* plasmine, tissue plasminogen activator, scuPA; Hemorheologic agents: *HAES, dextrans*
Abbreviations used:
ICA, internal carotid artery; MCA, middle cerebral artery; BA, basilar artery; VA, vertebral artery; SAE, subcortical arteriosclerotic encephalopathy; PTA, percutaneous transluminal angioplasty; RIND, reversible ischemic neurological deficit; PRIND, prolonged reversible ischemic neurological deficit; scuPA, single-chain urokinase plasminogen activator.
[b] In prevention of subsequent TIAs, stroke, or death. [c] "Minor stroke" includes RIND, PRIND, and recent completed stroke with minor sequelae.

siphon or MCA stenosis, intracranial vertebral artery or basilar artery stenosis. Because heparin prevents thrombus extension the intrinsic fibrinolytic mechanisms operate unopposed thereby augmenting the thrombolytic activity of tissue plasminogen activator (tPA) in vitro and in vivo [73].

Vitamin K Antagonists

Coumarins act as competitive inhibitors of vitamin K, blocking the final carboxylation step in the synthesis of the vitamin K dependent (extrinsic pathway) clotting factors II, VII, IX and X, and proteins C and S [74, 75]. Coumarin therapy is monitored by the prothrombin time (PT). Approximately one week or more of coumarin administration is required ot achieve a therapeutically significant reduction of the vitamin K dependent factors [76].

Coumarins have been used in long-term (3–6 months) treatment of presumed cardiac source thromboemboli. Its use in high-grade stenosis of the extra- and intracranial brain supplying arteries is not established by controlled trials [71, 77–79].

Antiplatelet Agents

Acetylsalicylic Acid (ASA)

ASA interacts with the thromboxane-prostacyclin (PGI_2) axis by inactivation of platelet-endothelium cyclooxygenase. By acetylation of cyclooxygenase, ASA blocks platelet thromboxane A_2 synthesis irreversibly [80–82], thereby inhibiting platelet aggregation and thromboxane A_2-mediated vasoconstriction. Low-dose ASA (80 mg per day) can irreversibly block cyclooxygenase in almost all circulating platelets while the endothelial production of PGI_2, which physiologically inhibits platelet aggregation, remains uninfluenced. Higher doses of ASA have been shown to block PGI_2 production in the endothelium [83].

Dipyridamole

Dipyridamole is a weak inhibitor of platelet aggregation. Inhibition of platelet phosphodiesterase, thereby increasing cytoplasmic cAMP, is probably responsible for the inhibition of platelet adhesion. It is possible that the antiplatelet properties of dipyridamole are caused by potentiation of the endogenous antiplatelet substance prostacyclin [84]. Dipyridamole acts synergistically with ASA to inhibit platelet function in vivo.

Sulfinpyrazone

Sulfinpyrazone appears to be a reversible inhibitor of thromboxane A_2, although the detailed mechanisms of antithrombotic action remain to be defined. High concentrations of sulfinpyrazone inhibit platelet aggregation induced by epinephrine or collagen in vitro. It can normalize a decreased platelet survival time associated with coronary artery disease and prosthetic heart valves [85].

Ticlopidine

The precise mechanism(s) of the platelet inhibitory effect(s) of ticlopidine are unknown. Ticlopidine has profound antiplatelet properties, which may result from an alteration of the platelet membrane affinity to activating stimuli. ADP-induced platelet aggregation is abolished, while thromboxane synthesis is not influenced [80].

Prostacyclin

Intravenous infusion of prostacyclin (PGI_2) has antiplatelet activity. Prostacyclin mediates vasodilatation and inhibits platelet aggregation. Elevated cyclic AMP-levels, which result from PGI_2-dependent stimulation of platelet adenylcyclase inhibit numerous platelet functions including platelet aggregation [80, 83, 86].

Antiplatelet agents, especially ASA, dipyridamole, and sulfinpyrazone prevent platelet adhesion and aggregation at the sites of arterial high flow and endothelial damage, thereby preventing or limiting platelet-mediated thrombus formation. They are advocated in preventing new thrombus formation, as well as growth of pre-existing thrombi due to additional platelet aggregation and have been used in the prevention of stroke following TIAs or previous stroke. Ticlopidine is the subject of an ongoing trial of the secondary prevention of stroke, that is, the prevention of a stroke subsequent to a signal stroke.

Interestingly, ASA is the only antiplatelet medication used in cerebrovascular occlusive disease that has shown a statistically significant therapeutic (preventive) effect in a number of major controlled studies [87, 88]. A survey on this topic has recently been published [80].

Neither the combination ASA/sulfinpyrazone nor the combination ASA/dipyridamole is more effective than ASA alone in the prophylactic management of TIAs in association with carotid artery disease [89]. The combination of ASA/coumarins is not recommended, since this combination has been reported to increase the risk of hemorrhage [90].

Fibrinolytic Agents

Endogenous fibrinolytic agents such as urokinase, tPA, and scuPa activate plasminogen to plasmin. Urokinase reacts with plasmin in the fluid phase thereby producing a systemic fibrinolytic state. Activated plasmin degrades both fibrin and fibrinogen. Additionally, fibrin and fibrinogen degradation products as well as the inactivation of factors V and VIII by urokinase/streptokinase produce a systemic anticoagulant state [91–93].

The fibrinolytic mechanisms of tPA and scuPA are described by Del Zoppo (this volume). It should be reemphasized that neither substance given in therapeutic doses generates a systemic anticoagulant state and they are therefore purported to have a diminished bleeding risk.

The exogenous agent streptokinase binds to plasminogen, thereby forming an active streptokinase-plasminogen complex. The complex can convert other molecules of plasminogen to plasmin. Streptokinase, like urokinase, produces a systemic fibrinolytic and anticoagulant effect.

Based on the mechanisms described above and despite the negative interpretation of uncontrolled early studies (survey: [94]), fibrinolytic agents, by analogy to coronary artery thrombosis, may be useful in the early recanalization and functional recovery of recent thromboembolic or thrombotic occlusions of major cranial vessels [95–98] when given systemically or locally. The incidence of the hemorrhagic complications during fibrinolytic therapy has been recently reviewed [94].

Other Agents

Activated Protein C

Activated protein C (APC) has indirect fibrinolytic properties in addition to its activity as a physiological inhibitor of factors V and VIII. APC results from the activation of protein C in the presence of endothelial cell thrombin-thrombomodulin complex. APC in human systems apparently inhibits circulating plasminogen activator inhibitor, thereby increasing the activity of tPA and local fibrinolytic activity. The anticoagulant potential of APC greatly exceeds its fibrinolytic capacity [99]. Whether APC will be of practical pharmacological value remains to be seen.

Defibrinating Enzymes

Defibrinating enzymes such as ancrod deplete fibrinogen by the formation of degradation products through induction of fibrin polymerization without activation of factor XIII. Ancrod also reduces blood viscosity [44].

Hemorheological Substances

Hemorheological (hemodilutional) substances such as hydroxyethyl starch and low molecular-weight dextrans have weak antithrombotic effects secondary to coating of platelets and the mechanical blockade of platelet aggregation [44, 100]. Additionally, hemorheological treatment increases blood flow in low-flow arterioles and by dilution lowers the fibrinogen level, which is usually augmented in high-viscosity states, thus additionally preventing thrombus formation. Very high viscosity levels have been reported in patients with a special subtype of cerebral microangiopathy (Binswanger's disease) [101]. Based on these mechanisms, hemorheological treatment is thought to be effective in hyperviscosity syndromes. However, the effectiveness of this approach has not been proven by controlled studies of acute stroke or completed stroke.

Conclusions

Thrombotic and thromboembolic events comprise the major cause of stroke. The known molecular aspects of platelet activation and aggregation, as well as of coagulation, leading to thrombus formation and extension, and the mechanisms of thrombus dissolution and fibrinolysis that lead to thromboembolism are all important to the occlusion of cerebral arteries which underlie cerebral ischemia. The degree and location of the region of cerebral ischemia is determined in part by the hemorheology of the individual cerebral circulation, and the presence of arterial collaterals. Peculiarities of the microanatomy of individual cerebral arterial segments may determine the characteristics and location of atheromata and thrombotic events. The use of antithrombotic agents in the treatment of thrombus-related cerebrovascular ischemia has been theoretically based upon the molecular aspects of thrombus formation outlined here. Based upon recent pathogenetic concepts of thrombotic stroke, the principles of thrombus formation and thrombolysis, and experimental and clinical data concerning the mechanisms of various antithrombotic agents, a differential treatment plan is proposed (Table 1). This proposal is necessarily limited, because, with the exception of the use of ASA in the secondary prevention of stroke, and coumarine prevention of cardiogenic emboli, no controlled clinical trials supporting the use of the agents listed have proven their efficacy.

References

1. Thomson AR, Harker LA (1983) Manual of hemostasis and thrombosis. FA Davis, Philadelphia
2. Penington DG (1981) Thrombopoiesis. In: Bloom AL, Thomas DP (eds) Haemostasis and thrombosis. Churchill Livingstone, Edinburgh, p 1
3. Ratnoff OD (1981) The role of haemostatic mechanisms. Clin Haematol 10:261–281
4. Toole JF (1985) Cerebrovascular disorders. Raven, New York
5. Mohr JP, Barnett HJM (1986) Classification of ischemic stroke. In: Barnett HJM, Mohr JP, Stein BM, Yatsu FM (eds) Stroke – pathophysiology, diagnosis and management. Churchill Livingstone, New York, p 281
6. Wolf PA, Kannel WB, McGee DL (1986) Epidemiology of stroke in North America. In: Barnett HJM, Mohr JP, Stein BM, Yatsu FM (eds) Stroke – pathophysiology, diagnosis and management. Churchill Livingstone, New York, p 19
7. Zülch KJ (1985) The cerebral infarct. Pathology, pathogenesis, and computed tomography. Springer, Berlin Heidelberg New York Tokyo
8. Zülch KJ (1981) Cerebrovascular pathology and pathogenesis as a basis of neuroradiological diagnosis. In: Diethelm L, Wende S (eds) Roentgendiagnosis of the central nervous system. Springer, Berlin Heidelberg New York, (Handbuch der medizinischen Radiologie, vol. XIV, part 1 A), pp 1–192
9. Mohr JP, Pessin MS (1986) Extracranial carotid artery disease. In: Barnett HJM, Mohr JP, Stein BM, Yatsu FM (eds) Stroke – pathophysiology, diagnosis and management. Churchill Livingstone, New York, p 293
10. Hachinski V, Norris JW (1985) The acute stroke. FA Davis, Philadelphia
11. Harker LA, Schwartz SM, Ross R (1982) Endothelium and arteriosclerosis. Clin Haematol 10:283–296
12. Miyakawa T, Sakuragowa N (1984) The cerebral vessels and thrombosis. Rinsho Ketsueki 25:1018–1026
13. Majno G, Joris I (1978) Endothelium: a review. Adv Exp Med 104:169–225
14. Zimmerman TS, Fierer J, Rothberger H (1977) Blood coagulation and the inflammatory response. Sem Hematol 14:391–408
15. Ginsberg MH, Henson PM (1978) Enhancement of platelet response to immune complexes and IgG aggregates by lipid A-rich bacterial lipopolysaccharides. J Exp Med 147:207–217
16. Zucker MB (1980) The functioning of blood platelet. Sci Am 242:86–103
17. Moncada S, Vane JR (1979) Arachidonic acid metabolites and the interactions between platelets and blood-vessel walls. N Engl J Med 300:1142–1147

18. Burstein SA, Harker LA (1981) Quantitative platelet disorders. In: Bloom AL, Thomas DP (eds) Haemostasis and thrombosis. Churchill Livingstone, Edinburgh, p 279
19. Kaplan AP (1978) Initiation of the intrinsic coagulation and fibrinolytic pathways of man: the role of surfaces, Hageman factor, prekallikrein, high molecular weight kininogen, and factor XI. Prog Hemostasis Thromb 4:127–175
20. Jackson CM, Nemerson Y (1980) Blood coagulation. Annu Rev Biochem 49:765–811
21. Gabes PC, Barnett HJM, Silver MD (1986) Cardiogenic stroke. In: Barnett HJM, Mohr JP, Stein BM, Yatsu FM (eds) Stroke – pathophysiology, diagnosis and management. Churchill Livingstone, New York, p 1085
22. Miletich JP, Jackson CM, Majerus PW (1978) Properties of the factor Xa binding site on human platelets. J Biol Chem 253:6908–6916
23. Baumgartner HR, Muggli R (1976) Adhesion and aggregation: morphological demonstration and quantitation in vivo and in vitro. In: Gordon JL (ed) Platelets in biology and pathology. Elsevier, New York, p 23
24. White JG, Clawson CC, Gerrard JM (1981) Platelet ultrastructure. In: Bloom AL, Thomas DP (eds) Haemostasis and thrombosis. Churchill Livingstone, Edinburgh, p 22
25. Berndt MC, Phillips DR (1981) Platelet membrane proteins: composition and receptor function. In: Gorden JL (ed) Platelets in biology and pathology, vol 2. Elsevier, New York, p 43
26. Gerrard JM, White JG (1978) Prostaglandins and thromboxanes: "middlemen" modulating platelet function in hemostasis and thrombosis. Prog Hemostasis Thromb 4:87–105
27. Marguerie GA, Plow EF (1981) Interaction of fibrinogen with its receptor: kinetics and effect of pH and temperature. Biochemistry 20:1074–1080
28. Bennett JS, Vilaire G (1979) Exposure of platelet fibrinogen receptors by ADP and epinephrine. J Clin Invest 64:1393–1401
29. Kaplan KL, Brockman MJ, Chernoff A, Lezznik GR, Drillings M (1979) Platelet alpha-granule proteins: Studies on release and subcellular localization. Blood 53:604–618
30. Morrison DC, Cochrane CG (1974) Direct evidence for Hagemann factor (factor XII) activation by bacterial lipopolysaccharides (endotoxins). J Exp Med 140:797–811
31. Sixma JJ (1981) Role of blood vessel, platelet and coagulation interactions in haemostasis. In: Bloom AL, Thomas DP (eds) Haemostasis and thrombosis. Churchill Livingstone, Edinburgh
32. Hermans J, McDonagh J (1982) Fibrin: structure and interactions. Semin Thromb Hemostasis 8:11–24
33. Mann KG, Tayler FB (1980) The Regulation of coagulation. Elsevier/North Holland, New York, p 145
34. Majerus PW et al. (1980) The formation of thrombin on platelet surface. In: Mann KG, Taylor FB (eds) The regulation of coagulation. Elsevier, New York, p 215
35. Collen D (1980) On the regulation and control of fibrinolysis. Thromb Haemostasis 43:77–89
36. Francis CW, Marder VJ, Barlow GH (1980) Plasmic degradation of crosslinked fibrin: characterization of new macromolecular soluble complexes and a model of their structure. J Clin Invest 66:1033–1043
37. Bachmann F, Kruithof IEKO (1984) Tissue plasminogen activator: chemical and physiological aspects. Semin Thromb Hemostasis 10:6–17
38. Harpel P (1982) Blood proteolytic enzyme inhibitors: their role in modulating blood coagulation and fibrinolytic pathways. In: Coleman RW et al. (eds) Hemostasis and thrombosis: basic principles and clinical practice. JP Lippincott, Philadelphia, p 738
39. Aoki N, Harpel PC (1984) Inhibitors of the fibrinolytic enzyme system. Semin Thromb Hemostasis 10:24–41
40. Clouse HL, Comp PC (1986) The regulation of hemostasis: the protein C system. N Engl J Med 314:1298–1304
41. Raish RJ, Hook JC (1986) Coagulopathy and stroke. In: Barnett HJM, Mohr JP, Stein BM, Yatsu FM (eds) Stroke – pathophysiology, diagnosis and management, Churchill Livingstone, New York, p 887
42. Rosenberg RD (1982) Heparin-antithrombin system. In: Coleman RW et al. (eds) Hemostasis and thrombosis: basic principles and clinical practice. JB Lippincott, Philadelphia, p 962
43. Marcus AJ (1979) The role of prostaglandins in platelet function. Prog Hematol 224:147–171
44. Dormandy JA (1981) Haemorheology and thrombosis. In: Bloom AL, Thomas DP (eds) Haemostasis and thrombosis. Churchill Livingstone, Edinburgh, p 1

45. Turitto VT, Miggli R, Baumgartner HR (1977) Physical factors influencing platelet deposition on subendothelium: importance of blood shear rate. NY Acad Sci USA 2:84–102
46. Goldsmith HL, Turitto VT (1986) Rheological aspects of thrombosis and haemostasis: basic principles and applications. Thrombosis Hemostas 55:415–435
47. Hellums JD, Brown CH (1977) Blood cell damage by mechanical forces. In: Hwang NHC, Normann NA (eds) Cardiovascular flow dynamics and measurements. University Park Press, Baltimore, p 799
48. Goldsmith HL, Yu SS, Marlow J (1975) Fluid mechanical stress and the platelet. Throm Diath Haemorrhag 34:32–41
49. Thomas DJ, Marshall J, Ross-Russel RW, Wetherley G, DuBoulay GH, Pearson R, Symon L, Zilkha E (1977) Effect of haematocrit on cerebral blood-flow in man. Lancet 2:941–943
50. Motomiya M, Karino T (1984) Flow patterns in the human carotid artery bifurcation. Stroke 15:50–56
51. Davies JA, Essien E, Cazenave J-P, Kinlough-Rathbone RL, Gent M, Mustard JF (1979) The influence of red blood cells on the effects of Aspirin and Sulphin pyrazone on platelet adherence to damaged rabbit aorta. Br J Haematol 42:283–291
52. Ringelstein EB, Zeumer H, Schneider R (1985) Der Beitrag der zerebralen Computertomographie zur Differentialtypologie und Differentialtherapie des ischaemischen Großhirninfarktes. Fortschr Neurol Psychiat 53:315
53. Fry DL (1976) Hemodynamic forces in atherosclerosis. In: Scheinberg P (ed) Cerebrovascular diseases. Raven Press, New York, p 77
54. Wolf N (1981) Thrombosis and atherosclerosis. In: Bloom AL, Thomas DP (eds) Haemostasis and thrombosis. Churchill Livingstone, Edinburgh, p 1
55. Gryglewski RJ (1980) Prostaglandins, platelets and atherosclerosis. CRC Crit Rev Biochem 7:291–338
56. Garcia JH, Cox JV, Oludgins WR (1971) Ultrastructure of the microvasculature in experimental cerebral infarction. Acta Neuropathol (Berl) 18:273–285
57. Nadjmi M, Ratzka M (1981) Normale Anatomie der cerebralen Arterien. In: Diethelm L, Wende S (eds) Roentgendiagnosis of the central nervous system. Springer, Berlin Heidelberg New York (Handbuch der medizinischen Radiologie, vol XIV, part 1 A), pp 327
58. Duvernoy HM (1978) Human brainstem vessels. Springer, Berlin Heidelberg New York
59. Van der Eecken HM, Adams RD (1959) The anatomy and functional significance of the meningeal arterial anastomoses of the human brain. J Neuropathol Exp Neurol 12:132–141
60. Uhle G, Kolkmann FW (1972) Normale und pathologische Anatomie des Hirngefäßsytems – pathologische Anatomie. In: Gaenshirt H (ed) Der Hirnkreislauf. Physiologie – Pathologie – Klinik. Thieme, Stuttgart, p 45
61. Moossy J (1984) Anatomy and physiology of the vertebrobasilar system. In: Berguer R, Bauer RB (eds) Vertebrobasilar arterial occlusive disease. Raven Press, New York
62. Nag S (1984) Cerebral endothelial surface charge in hypertension. Acta Neuropathol (Berl) 63:276–281
63. Fisher CM (1969) The arterial lesions underlying lacunes. Acta Neuropathol (Berl) 12:1–15
64. Mohr JP (1982) Lacunes. Stroke 13:3–11
65. Hirsh P (1986) Anticoagulant and platelet antiaggregant agents. In: Barnett HJM, Mohr JP, Stein BM, Yatsu FM (eds) Stroke – pathophysiology, diagnosis, and management Churchill Livingstone, New York, p 925
66. Barrowcliffe TW, Thomas DP (1981) Antithrombin III and heparin. In: Bloom AL, Thomas DP (eds) Haemostasis and thrombosis, Churchill Livingstone, Edinburgh, p 1
67. Rosenberg RD (1976) Actions and interactions of antithrombin and heparin. N Engl J Med 292:146–151
68. Lollar P, Owen WG (1980) Clearance of thrombin from circulation in rabbits by high affinity binding sites on endothelium. J Clin Invest 66:1222–1230
69. Thaler E, Lechner K (1981) Antithrombin III deficiency and thromboembolism. Clin Haematol 10:369–390
70. Brandt JT, Triplett DA (1981) Laboratory monitoring of heparin. Effect of reagents and instruments on the activated partial thromboplastin time. Am J Clin Pathol 76(Suppl):530–537
71. Millikan CH, McDowell FH (1981) Treatment of progressing stroke. Stroke 12:397–409
72. Marshall J (1976) The management of cerebrovascular diseases. Blackwell, Oxford, p 150

73. Cercek B, Lew AS, Hod H, Yano J, Reedy NKN, Ganz W (1986) Enhancement of thrombolysis with tissue-type plasminogen activator by pretreatment with heparin. Circulation 74:583–587
74. Breckenridge A (1978) Oral anticoagulant drugs: pharmacokinetic aspects Semin Hematol 15:19–26
75. O'Reilly RA (1976) Vitamin K and other oral anticoagulant drugs. Annu Rev Med 24:249–261
76. Loeliger EA, (1979) The optimal therapeutic range in oral anticoagulation history and proposal. Thromb Haemostasis 42:1141–1152
77. Baker RN, Broward JA, Fang HC, Fisher CM, Groch SN, Heyman A, Karp HR, McDevitt E, Scheinberg P, Schwartz W, Toole JF (1962) Anticoagulant therapy in cerebral infarction. Neurology 12:823–835
78. Furlan AJ, Cavalier SJ, Hobbs RE, Weinstein MA, Modic MI (1982) Hemorrhage and anticoagulation after nonseptic embolic brain infarction. Neurology 32:280–282
79. Cerebral Embolism Study Group (1984) Immediate anticoagulant of embolic stroke: Brain hemorrhage and management options. Stroke 15:779–789
80. Harker LA (1986) Antiplatelet drugs in the management of patients with thrombotic disorders. Sem Thromb Hemost 12:134–155
81. Roth GJ, Majerus PW (1975) The mechanism of the effect of aspirin on human platelet. I. Acetylation of a particulate fraction protein. J Clin Invest 56:624–632
82. Majerus PW, Miletich JP (1978) Relationships between platelets and coagulation factors in haemostasis. Annu Rev Med 29:41
83. Burch JW, Stanford N, Majerus PW (1978) Inhibition of platelet prostaglandin synthetase by oral aspirin. J Clin Invest 61:314–319
84. Smith JB (1981) Dipyridamole may be more effective with sodium salicylate than with aspirin. Am Heart J 101:686–687
85. Kelton JG (1983) Antiplatelet agennts: rationale and results. In: Harker LA, Zimmerman TS (eds) Clinics in hematology, vol 12, Platelet disorders. Saunders. London, pp 318ff
86. Burch JW, Majerus PW (1979) The role of prostaglandins in platelet function. Semin Hematol 16:196–207
87. Fields WS, Lemak NA, Frankowski RF, Hardy FJ (1978) Controlled trial of aspirin in cerebral ischemia. Part II: Surgial Group. Stroke 9:309–319
88. Sorensen PS, Pedersen H, Marquardsen J, Peterson H, Hellberg A, Simonsen S, Andersen LA (1983) Acetylsalicylic acid in the prevention of stroke in patients with reversible cerebral ischemic attacks: a Danish cooperative study. Stroke 14:15–22
89. The Canadian Cooperative Study Group: A randomized trial of aspirin and sulfinpyrazone in threatened stroke. N Engl J Med 299:53–59
90. Chesebro JH, Fuster V, Elveback LR, McGoon DC, Pluth JR, Puga FJ, Wallace RB, Danielson GK, Orszulak TA, Piehler JM, Schaff HV (1983) Trial of combined warfarin plus dipyridamole or aspirin therapy in prosthetic heart valve replacement: danger of aspirin compared with dipyridamole. Am J Cardiol 51:1537–1541
91. Castellino FJ (1984) Biochemistry of human plasminogen. Semin Thromb Hemostasis 10:18–23
92. Kakkar VV, Scully MF (1978) Thrombolytic therapy. Br Med Bull 34:191–199
93. Sharma GVRK, Cella G, Parish AF, Sasahara AA (1982) Drug therapy: thrombolytic therapy. N Engl J Med 306:1268–1276
94. Del Zoppo GJ, Zeumer H, Harker LA (1986) Thrombolytic therapy in acute stroke: possibilities and hazards. Stroke 17:595–607
95. Zeumer H (1985) Survey of progress: Vascular recanalizing techniques in interventional neuroradiology. J Neurol 231:287–294
96. Zeumer H, Hacke W, Kolmann HL, Poeck K (1982) Lokale Fibrinolysetherapie bei Basilaristhrombose. Dtsch Med Wochenschr 107:728–731
97. Zeumer H, Hacke W, Ringelstein EF (1983) Local intraarterial thrombolysis in vertebrobasilar thromboembolic diseases. Am J Neuroradiol 4:401–404
98. Del Zoppo GJ, Hacke W (1987) Fibrinolytische Therapie bei ischämischen Hirninfarkten. Dtsch Med Wschr 112:603–608
99. Comp PC, Esmon CT (1981) Generation of fibrinolytic activity by infusion of activated protein C into dogs. J Clin Invest 68:1221–1228
100. Wood JH, Kee DB (1986) Clinical hemorheology of stroke and hemodilution. In: Barnett HJM, Mohr JP, Stein BM, Yatsu FM (eds) Stroke – pathophysiology, diagnosis and management. Churchill-Livingstone, New York, p 97
101. Schneider R, Ringelstein EB, Zeumer H, Kiesewetter H, Jung F (1987) The role of plasma hyperviscosity in subcortical arteriosclerotic encephalopathy (Binswanger's disease). J Neurol 234:67–73
102. Harker LA, Fuster V (1986) J Am Coll Cardiol 8:21B–32B

Computed Tomography Patterns of Brain Infarctions as a Pathogenetic Key

H. ZEUMER [1] and E. B. RINGELSTEIN [1]

Introduction

Traditionally, differentiation of patients suffering from ischemic strokes was based on clinical findings and the course of the disease. Categories such as transient ischemic attacks (TIA), prolonged reversible ischemic neurological deficit (PRIND), and completed stroke have been used as major criteria for stroke classification and consequently for therapeutic decision-making. Before CT became available, and when angiography was still widely used as the basic diagnostic tool for imaging of cerebrovascular disease, virtually any type and degree of carotid lesion could be correlated with numerous hemispheric ischemic events. This was also true of cerebrovascular accidents and associated arterial lesions within the vertebrobasilar system. Hemodynamic mechanisms were thought to be the major factors in the pathophysiology of stroke.

In recent decades, however, numerous concepts related to stroke pathogenesis have had to be revised. Firstly, hemodynamically induced, i.e., watershed and low-flow, infarctions were found to be relatively rare and to occur as a result of very tight, often multiple stenoses and occlusions [22–24,34] – but *not* medium-grade lesions or syncopes. Secondly, the role of low-degree carotid stenoses as a source of emboli had probably been overestimated. It should be noted in this context that cardiac emboli, which make up about 40% of embolic strokes [20], can easily pass nonstenosing and medium-sized ICA lesions, although not tight stenoses and occlusions. Thirdly, high-grade stenoses often have thrombotic tails floating downstream which may easily act as large emboli leading to severe arterio-arterial embolic strokes [23] (see Hacke et al., this volume).

Dramatic methodological improvements have also occurred both in detection of brain infarctions and in evaluation of the underlying arterial lesions. Angiography is no longer a neuroangiological screening method. Its application requires ample justification for the neuroradiologist to use such an invasive procedure. This has come to be of utmost concern since extracranial continuous-wave Doppler, pulsed transcranial ultrasound, and B-mode imaging have enabled us to quantify and monitor brain artery lesions noninvasively. These techniques also permit us to define the hemodynamic relevance of arterial stenoses and occlusions (see Ringelstein, this volume). Cerebral angiography is still necessary in order to demonstrate the precise morphology of a vascular lesion and to varify *distal* branch occlusions of the intracranial arteries.

---

[1] Department of Neurology, Klinikum RWTH, University Hospital, D-5100 Aachen, FRG

Advantage of Simultaneous Brain-Morphological and Angiological Studies In Vivo

Before the advent of CT the pathogenesis of stroke could only be studied retrospectively by neuropathologists on the basis of post-mortem findings. It was always a questionable procedure to relate in vivo angiographic findings to post-mortem brain morphology during necropsy, but this was the best available approach at that time. Zülch [35], for instance, presented a classification of brain infarctions differentiating between territorial, watershed and terminal supply area infarctions. However, due to the above-mentioned methodological shortcomings, hemodynamic aspects in the pathogenesis of brain infarctions were totally overestimated [25], presumably because recanalized emboli could no longer be found during necropsy. The *simultaneous* analysis of clinical and angiological findings, on the one hand, and brain infarctions, on the other was not possible until CT made brain pathology visible in vivo.

Typology of Brain Infarctions

Small-Vessel Disease

Fisher [10, 11], on the basis of post-mortem and clinical findings, taught us the importance of occlusive disease in the small intracerebral perforating arteries for the pathogenesis of stroke in the elderly. He demonstrated that lacunes occur due to segmental arteriosclerotic occlusions of the long, penetrating intracerebral arteries. These arterial lesions lead to small ovoid or pea-shaped cavities which are 2 – 10 mm in diameter. The infarctions are located within the irrigated areas of the thin (20 – 100 μg) but very long, penetrating vessels, i.e., the basal ganglia, the brainstem and, less frequently, the periventricular white matter (Fig. 1 a). Lacunar stroke patients represent 23% – 30% of the cases in stroke populations [9, 17].

With the help of CT, however, it was learned that clinical signs of lacunar strokes are unreliable with respect to the underlying type of brain lesion. Lacunar syndromes may be related to processes of quite different etiology. These may be typical lacunes within the basal ganglia, but also small cortical infarctions of embolic origin, as well as small low-flow-induced white-matter lesions or small bleedings [5, 18, 19, 28]. On the other hand, CT also taught us that lacunes are even more frequent than originally thought and are present in approximately one-third of all stroke patients if one includes the clinically silent ones as well [9, 15, 24]. Lacunar infarctions only represent the tip of an iceberg, as it were, in that they are indicative of a generalized small-vessel disease [7, 30].

The arteries involved in small-vessel disease cannot be visualized angiographically. With the help of CT, however, we are able to demonstrate the sequelae of small-vessel disease and to make the diagnosis indirectly by evaluating the lacunes and ischemic white-matter encephalopathy [19, 24, 28, 31 – 33]. But even with the help of MRI techniques [8, 13] it is not yet possible to demonstrate every single small lacune in the individual brain. From a practical point of view, this is also

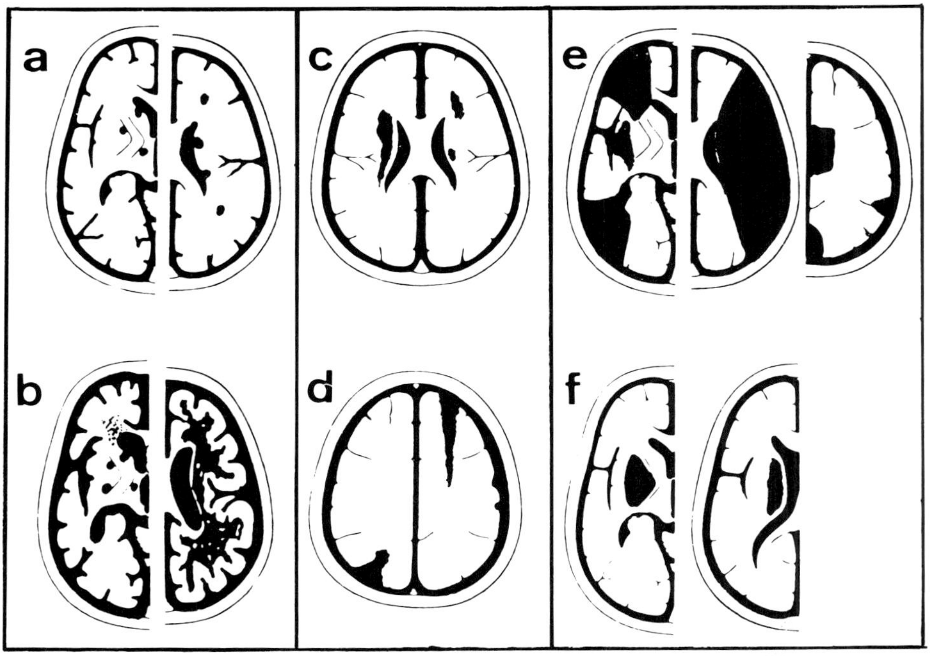

Fig. 1a–f. Different patterns of infarctions on CT.
a, b Cerebral microangiopathy is indicated by either multiple lacunar infarctions of typical size and site, i.e., lacunar state **(a)**, and/or by additional increased x-ray translucency of the periventricular white matter **(b)**. The latter type of brain damage is called subcortical arteriosclerotic encephalopathy (SAE) (Binswanger's type). **c, d** Low-flow induced infarctions occur either strictly subcortically in the periventricular white matter as so-called terminal supply area infarctions **(c)**, or as combined cortical and subcortical lesions between the large territories of the pial arteries **(d)**. These latter, interterritorial infarctions are also called watershed infarctions or borderzone infarctions. A small terminal supply area infarction (**c**, *right side*) cannot be unequivocally distinguished from a single lacune. **e, f** Territorial infarctions are restricted to the territory of large pial arteries and their branches. The cortical type **(e)** shows lesions of the anterior, insular, posterior main branches of the MCA (*left side*), total infarction of the MCA territory (*middle*), or infarctions in the territory of the pericallosal artery, posterior cerebral artery, and a very distal branch of the middle cerebral artery (*right side*). **f** subcortical version of a territorial infarction; the lesion involves a large area of the basal ganglia (*left side*), clearly exceeding the size of lacunes and, simultaneously, the terminal supply area of the lenticulostriate arteries (*right side*). This large extension of the infarction without involvement of the cortex is pathognomonic. (Modified from Ringelstein et al. [23])

not necessary. It is the presence of lacunes and ischemic white-matter encephalopathy per se, and not the quantitative aspect of the ischemic brain damage, which is indicative of this particular type of cerebrovascular disease [24, 33].

For proper reading of CT images, one should consider that lacunes are not sufficiently defined by means of their diameter, which ranges from 2–15 mm. The term lacune implies a certain pathogenesis of the lesion, namely the thrombotic occlusion of a single, long, perforating artery due to lipohyalinosis, as initially described by Fisher (1969) and by DeReuck and Vander Eecken (1976). The

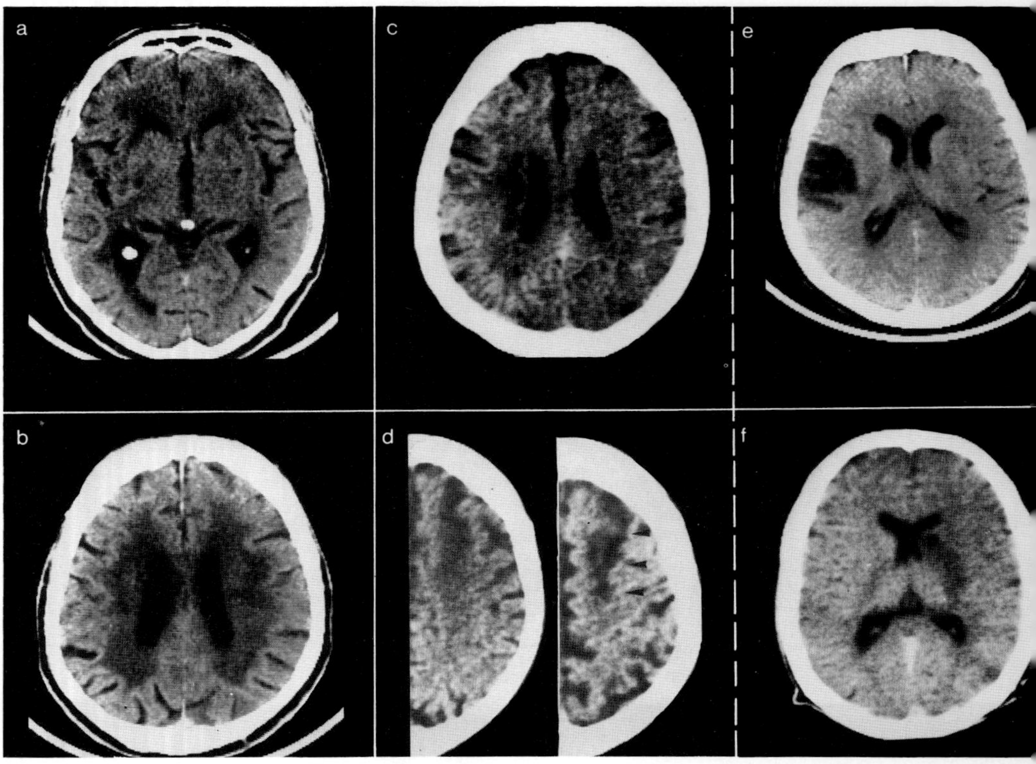

Fig. 2a–f. Illustrative cases of different brain infarctions demonstrated on CT images. **a, b** Typical CT with subcortical arteriosclerotic encephalopathy with lacunar state (**a**) and periventricular ischemic white-matter disease (**b**). **c** Right-side terminal supply area infarction. **d** Typical frontal watershed infarction. **e** Typical territorial infarction of the medial main branch of the MCA. **f** Typical large ganglionic infarction, i.e., striatocapsular infarction with involvement of the lentiform and caudate nuclei and the internal capsule. **a, b** represent small-vessel disease; **c–f** show large vessel disease. (Modified after Zeumer and Hacke [34])

diagnosis can only be made if lesions of typical size are seen in areas which are supplied by these deep, long perforators. Predilection sites have already been mentioned (Fig. 2a). Lesions of lacunar size, however, may also occur in the white matter [9, 24, 32]. From CT morphological studies in large series of patients suffering from lacunar states [28, 32] and from pathoanatomical findings [7] we know that lacunar infarctions rarely occur in the periventricular white matter. On the other hand, low-flow infarctions in the terminal supply area of the perforating long arteries of the centra semiovalia are not an infrequent phenomenon and have a similar appearance to lacunes (Fig. 1c, 2c). The therapeutic consequences of low-flow induced brain lesions, however, are completely different from those of lacunes, as will be outlined below.

Due to initial edema, recent lacunes may appear much larger than their residual defect. The latter should not exceed 15 mm. It is not judicious to apply the term "giant lacune" to relatively large infarctions restricted to the basal ganglia, since a middle cerebral artery occlusion may be the underlying pathology with a concomitant occlusion of several lenticulostriate arteries at their mouths (see below) [1, 23, 24, 27, 32]. In general, one should not overemphasize the term lacune in doubtful cases, particularly in solitary small white-matter infarctions. Additional clinical information, i.e., focal neurological signs, course of the stroke and Doppler ultrasound findings, both extracranial and intracranial (or even angiography), will help to define the true nature of the lesion.

Using high-resolution CT scanners hemispheric lesions are rarely missed. This is why patients with persistent neurological deficits who have an obviously normal CT are then highly suspect of a strategic vascular lesion in the hind-brain, too small to be visible on CT. Brainstem strokes occur more often than is generally believed, at least as often as hemispheric strokes. This clinical experience is confirmed by the sharp increase in the incidence of pathologic findings in the posterior fossa with the introduction of MRI [13].

It is quite remarkable that both ultrasound studies and pathoanatomical findings reveal the frequent occurrence of a *dilatative* type of arteriosclerosis within the *large* vessels in patients with simultaneous small-vessel disease. *Occlusive* large-vessel disease, by contrast, is a relatively rare event in these patients [9, 15]. This is also true of a more severe manifestation of small-vessel disease, namely the *subcortical arteriosclerotic encephalopathy* of Binswanger's type. This condition has been described pathoanatomically by Olzewski [21] and by Jellinger and Neumayr [16]. Recently this condition has very frequently been identified with the help of CT [24, 31, 33] (Figs. 1 b, 2 b) and has been further studied by means of clinical and electrophysiological techniques [3, 14, 31, 33].

Infarctions Indicating Large-Vessel Disease

It seems justifiable to divide the stroke population into those who suffer predominantly from small-vessel disease and those who mainly have obstructed lesions of the large extracranial and/or intracranial arteries, i.e. large vessel-disease – despite the obvious existence of mixed types [9, 24]. The reason for this division is less theoretical than practical: these two types differ totally in their pathogenesis and, consequently, in the diagnostic and therapeutic implications [15, 23, 24, 32]. Firstly, patients with large-vessel disease are candidates for vascular surgery or may be treated with antiplatelet agents or anticoagulants. By contrast, those with generalized intracerebral arteriosclerotic small-vessel disease do not benefit from the surgical removal of atherosclerotic carotid plaques, and anticoagulants may even have deleterious effects on them. Secondly, patients suffering from small-vessel disease often have hemorheological abnormalities and arterial hypertension, as well as diabetes mellitus. These should be treated by means of conservative measures [26].

With the help of CT therapeutic and diagnostic decisions may be facilitated not only in patients who display the pattern of small-vessel disease but also in those with large infarctions of the territorial or low-flow type (Fig. 1 c–f). *Territorial infarctions* are visible on CT either as purely cortical or combined cortical *and* subcortical defects of wedge-like, trapezoid, or half-moon-like shapes which are restricted to the territory of the supplying pial artery, i.e., the main cerebral arteries or their large, leptomeningeal branches (Figs. 1e, 1f, 2e). These lesions occur as a result of thromboembolic or, much more rarely, vasculitic arterial occlusions. If such a brain lesion is associated with normal ultrasound and/or angiographic findings, a cardiogenic, transient or distal embolic arterial occlusion is highly probable. If transcranial Doppler ultrasound reveals hyperperfusion of the main supplying artery of the infarcted area, spontaneous recanalization of this artery has taken place.

The final extent of the infarction within the affected vascular territory depends strongly on the recruitment and capacity of the collateral pathways, i.e., the leptomeningeal anastomoses and the configuration of the circle of Willis. It is also important how far distally emboli lodge within the vascular tree, with the more distal occlusions leading to smaller infarctions.

A very special situation is presented in patients with a segmental and often transient occlusion of the stem of the MCA [1, 23, 24, 27, 32]. Emboli at this site will occlude several if not all of the mouths of the lenticulostriate arteries. The latter are true endarteries, and their blockage will lead to large infarctions including both the basal ganglia *and* the terminal supply area of the "perforators" within the periventricular white matter (Figs. 1f, 2f). This type of infarction (i.e., lentiform nucleus infarction [23], striatocapsular infarction [1], large ganglionic infarction [20]) represents the subcortical version of a territorial infarction which also suggests a thromboembolic pathogenesis of the stroke due to macroangiopathy of the middle or anterior cerebral artery.

In patients with complete MCA occlusion, a large cortical infarction of the affected hemispherical cortex will occur only if the collateral blood supply via the leptomeningeal anastomoses is insufficient. This is usually the case in persistent acute embolic occlusions with apposition thrombus formation. We conclude that patients with large basal ganglia infarctions without involvement of the cortex either have stenosed but not occluded MCAs, or early recanalization due to spontaneous or therapeutically induced fibrinolysis has occurred. Also possible is recruitment of an excellent collateralization of the total MCA territory due to a gradual development of this lesion [24].

A small territorial infarction due to peripheral embolization may not be recognized clinically. In these cases with pseudo-asymptomatic ICA stenoses, CT findings may help to decide whether the patient should undergo carotid endarterectomy. A territorial type of brain infarction, even of lacunar size, is always highly suggestive of local arterio-arterial or cardiogenic embolization. By contrast, true lacunes are never situated in the cortex and, obviously, do not occur due to embolism of the brain.

Multiple territorial infarctions, particularly if they occur bilaterally, suggest cardiac embolism or vasculitis as the underlying mechanism of stroke, even if extracranial arterial lesions are also present. In conclusion, every CT demonstration of a territorial type of infarction, regardless of size, requires further careful neurological and laboratory investigations of the pathogenesis of the lesion. Carotid bifurcations and the heart are the most frequent sources of embolism.

One of two types of *low-flow infarctions* which can be differentiated on CT images (Figs. 1c, d, 2c, d) is the so-called *terminal supply area infarction* (Figs. 1c, 2c). This kind of lesion occurs exclusively as subcortical infarction in the white matter at and above the corpus callosum level, strictly sparing both the cortex and the basal ganglia [23, 24].

Borderzone or watershed infarctions [12, 24, 29, 34], on the other hand, are interterritorial lesions which always involve the cerebral cortex. They appear either as parasagittal lesions extending from the frontal to the parietal cortex (Fig. 1 d, right side; Fig. 2 d) or as parietooccipital defects within the borderzone of the temporoparietooccipital triangle (Fig. 1 d, left side).

Low-flow induced, subcortical white-matter infarctions range in size from 5 mm to nearly complete softening of the centrum semiovale. The smaller ones should not be confused with lacunes. Careful sonographic or angiographic examination usually demonstrates multiple and high-grade arterial lesions [22, 23, 24] such as stenotic or hypoplastic segments within the circle of Willis combined with severe stenoses or occlusions of the extracranial vessels. Occasionally, however, low-flow infarctions may also be found without any of these vascular obstructions. This is particularly true of the small subcortical type. They can be explained by temporary occlusion of a large pial artery or transient high-grade stenosis. Hemodynamically induced infarctions are generally found in the case of vasospasm due to subarachnoid hemorrhage but can also be induced by vasculitis and by rapidly recanalized emboli.

In a prospective study of 28 stroke patients, however, with proven cardiogenic embolism as the underlying stroke mechanism without any stenotic or occlusive lesions of the extracranial or intracranial large arteries, not a single case was observed with the typical low-flow pattern. All of these patients revealed the territorial type of brain damage (Fig. 3).

Infarctions in the Posterior Circulation

Due to their small size and infrequent appearance, lacunar infarctions of the brainstrem and cerebellum are rarely visible on CT images. But these will be demonstrated more often as soon as MRI becomes a routine method [13]. A pathogenetic analysis of the patterns of infarctions in the brainstem, particularly of the pons and mesencephalon, is by far more difficult than one in the hemispheres. One of the reasons for this is that pontine infarctions, if visible at all, are small and often not larger than lacunes. In this case, only the outer delineation of the infarction allows a further differentiation. While lacunes are ovoid or ball-shaped, small territorial infarctions of the pontine branches (rami ad pontem) are triangular or wedge-shaped (Fig. 4). Whereas the first indicate vertebrobasilar microangiopathy, the latter probably occur due to macroangiopathy of the basilar artery [4].

Due to their large size, infarctions in the territories of the cerebellar arteries are easier to detect. They are of major clinical interest, as they may lead to acute compression of the fourth ventricle and hydrocephalus. The indication for surgery is based on both clinical and CT findings. CT examinations must be performed repeatedly during the first week after stroke onset [6].

The early diagnosis of basilar artery thrombosis relies exclusively on clinical and angiographical (or ultrasound) findings. As soon as extended brainstem or cerebellar infarctions have become visible on CT, an irreversible and prognostical-

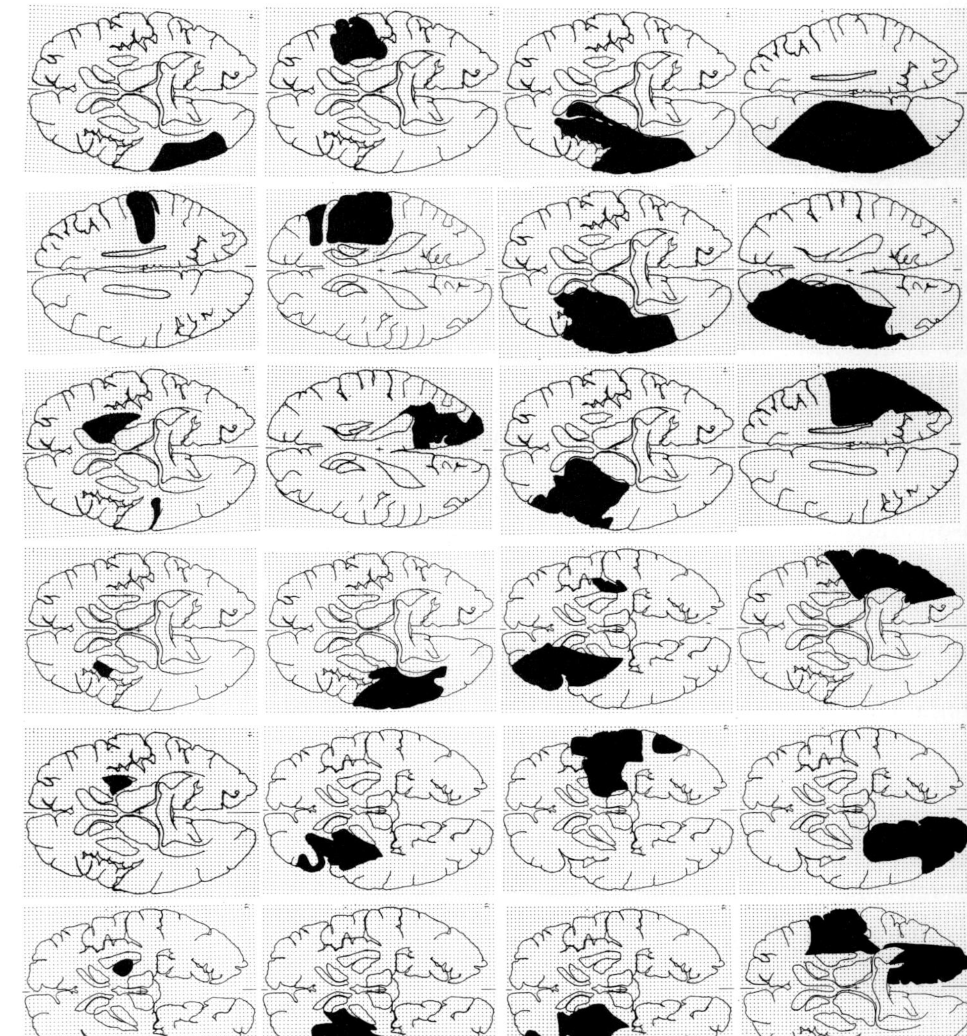

Fig. 3. Brain infarctions in patients with proven cardiogenic embolism. Brain slices with the largest extension of infarction(s) are shown, each slice representing one patient. These are the results of the first 28 patients of a prospective study. Each lesion was of the territorial type of infarction, except for the first case where the infarction could not be categorized. (From Ringelstein and Koschorke, unpublished data)

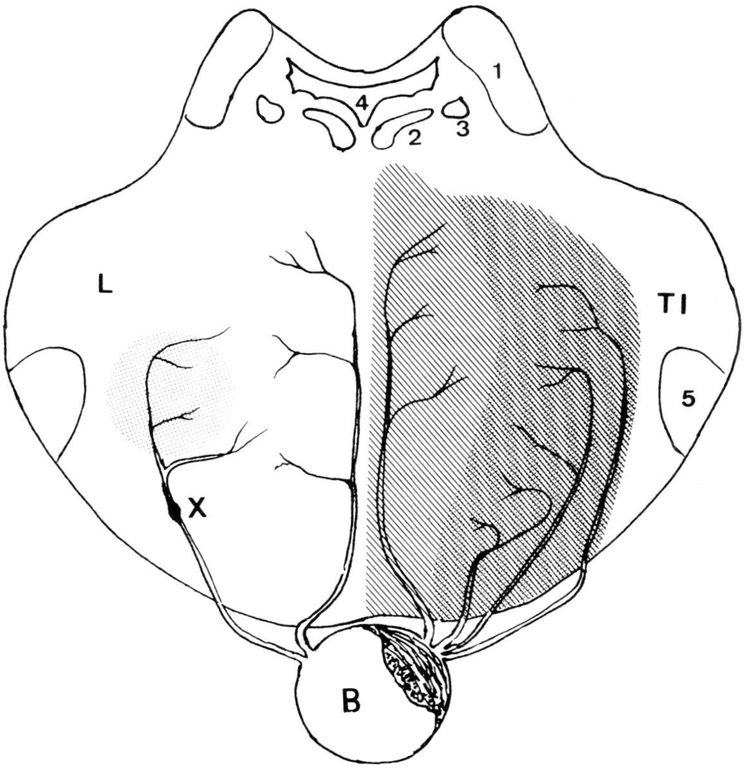

Fig. 4. Schematic drawing of various pontine infarctions and their underlying vascular lesions. A typical ovoid lacunar infarction is visible (*left side*) which occurred due to an occlusive microangiopathic process (*x*) of one of the perforating arteries (rami ad pontem). The wedge-shaped infarction (*right side*) represents the territory of the paramedian and short circumflexor branches, respectively, of the rami ad pontem. The whole territories are infarcted. The underlying vascular lesion is an atherothrombotic, i.e., macroangiopathic, process within the basilar artery (*B*). *1*, Pedunculus cerebellaris superior; *2*, fasciculus longitudinalis medialis; *3*, locus coeruleus; *4*, fourth ventricle; *5*, trigeminal nerve; *L*, lacune; *TI*, territorial infarction (compare also Caplan and Rosenbaum 1975, p. 602, Fig. 1)

ly poor state of the disease has been reached [2]. At such time fibrinolytic therapy would no longer make sense.

Conclusions

From a diagnostic point of view, the small brain infarctions visible on CT are the most delicate ones. However, these are important with respect to their clinical impact. To detect such lesions, it is necessary to perform careful CT studies with appropriate and consistent measuring and with photographic parameters which also include the apical slices of the brain. Sometimes a repeated CT is necessary to prove the reproducibility of a small infarction and to rule out noise interference.

Although MRI offers no specific advantage in the diagnosis of infarctions per se, this method will improve the detection of small low-flow induced lesions within the terminal supply areas and lacunes, as well as that of small territorial infarctions within the brainstem. Particularly in small brain infarctions, the simple description of size and location of the infarcted area is clinically insufficient. The diagnostician should add more pathogenetically relevant data. This is only possible, however, if the close association of distinct brain infarctions with different types of cerebrovascular and cardiac diseases is considered. Here the diagnostic impact of CT in stroke patients is considerable. Typical morphological patterns can be identified and may give reliable clues as to the pathogenesis of brain infarction. This will automatically lead to adequate therapeutic strategies.

References

1. Bladin PF, Berkovic SF (1984) Striatocapsular infarction: Large infarcts in the lenticulostriate arterial territory. Neurology 34:1423–1430
2. Brückmann H, Ferbert A, del Zoppo GJ, Hacke W, Ringelstein EB, Zeumer H (1986) The acute vertebral-basilar thrombosis: angiological-clinical comparison and therapeutic implications. Acta Radiol 369:38–42 (Suppl)
3. Caplan LR, Rosenbaum AE (1975) Role of cerebral angiography in vertebro-basilar occlusive disease. J Neurol Neurosurg Psychiat 38:601–612
4. Caplan LR, Schoene W (1978) Clinical features of subcortical arteriosclerotic encephalopathy (Binswanger Disease). Neurology 28:1206–1215
5. Chokroverty CS, Rubino FA, Haller C (1977) Pure motor hemiplegia due to cerebral cortical infarction. Arch Neurol 34:93–95
6. Cioffi FA, Bernini FP, Punzo A, Avanzo RD (1985) Surgical management of acute cerebellar infarction. Acta Neurochirurgica 74:105–112
7. De Reuck J, Vander Eecken H (1976) The arterial angioarchitecture in lacunar state. Acta Neurol Belg 76:142–149
8. De Witt LD (1986) Clinical use of nuclear magnetic resonance imaging in stroke. Stroke 17:328–331
9. Ferbert A, Zeumer H, Ringelstein EB (1985) Dopplersonographische Befunde beim ischämischen Hirninfarkt unterschiedlicher Pathogenese. Akt. Neurol. 12:153–157
10. Fisher CM (1969) The arterial lesions underlying lacunes. Acta Neuropathol. 12:1–15
11. Fisher CM (1982) Lacunar strokes and infarcts: a review. Neurology 32:871–876
12. Fisher M, McQuillen JB (1981) Bilateral cortical border-zone infarction. Arch Neurol 38:62–63
13. Fox AJ, Bogousslavsky J, Carey LS, Barnett HJM, Vinitski H, Karlik SJ, Vinuela F, Pelz DM, Hachinski V (1986) Magnetic resonance imaging of small medullary infarctions. AJNR 7:229–233
14. George AE, DeLeon M, Gentes CI, Miller J, London E, Budzilovich G, Ferris S, Chase N (1984) Leukoencephalopathy of aging: CT clinical-neuropathologic study of brain lucencies. AJNR 5:678
15. Guse F, Weiller C, Brückmann H, Ringelstein EB (1987) Zur Abhängigkeit des Hirninfarktrisikos vom Schweregrad okkludierender Karotis interna-Läsionen. Nervenarzt 58 (in press)
16. Jellinger K, Neumayr E (1964) Progressive subkortikale vaskuläre Encephalopathie Binswanger: eine klinisch-neuropathologische Studie. Arch Psychiat Nervenkr 285:523–554
17. Mohr JP (1977) Sensorimotor stroke due to thalamocapsular ischemia. Arch Neurol 34:739–741
18. Mori E, Tabuchi J, Yamadori A (1985) Lacunar syndrome due to intracerebral hemorrhage. Stroke 16:454–459
19. Nelson RF, Pullicino R, Kendall BE, Marshall J (1980) Computed tomography in patients presenting with lacunar syndromes. Stroke 11:256–261

20. Olsen TS, Skriver C, Herning M (1985) Cause of cerebral infarction in the carotid territory: its relation to the size and the location of the infarct and to the underlying vascular lesion. Stroke 16:459–466
21. Olszewski J (1962) Subcortical arteriosclerotic encephalopathy. World Neurol 3:359–364
22. Rodda RA, Path FRC (1986) The arterial patterns associated with internal carotid and cerebral infarcts. Stroke 17:69–75
23. Ringelstein EB, Zeumer H, Angelou D (1983) The pathogenesis of strokes from internal carotid artery occlusion. Diagnostic and therapeutical implications. Stroke 14:867–875
24. Ringelstein EB, Zeumer H, Schneider R (1985) Der Beitrag der zerebralen Computertomographie zur Differentialtypologie und Differentialtherapie des ischämischen Großhirninfarktes. Fortsch Neurol Psychiat 9:315–354
25. Schneider M (1953) Durchblutung und Sauerstoffversorgung des Gehirns. Verh Dtsch Ges Kreisl Forsch 19:3–25
26. Schneider R, Körber N, Zeumer H, Kiesewetter H, Ringelstein EB, Brockmann M (1985) The haemorheological features of lacunar strokes. J Neurol 232:357–359
27. Taneda M, Shimada N, Tsuchiya T (1985) Transient neurological deficits due to embolic occlusion and reopening of the cerebral arteries. Stroke 16:522–534
28. Weisberg LA (1982) Lacunar infarcts: clinical and computed tomographic correlations. Arch Neurol 39:37–40
29. Wodarz R (1980) Watershed infarctions and computed tomography. A topographical study in cases with stenosis or occlusion of the carotid artery. Neuroradiology 19:245–248
30. Zeumer H, Hacke W (1982) Zur Frage der Multiinfarktdemenz unter besonderer Berücksichtigung computertomographischer Befunde. Fortsch Neurol Psychiat 50:366–367
31. Zeumer H, Hacke W, Hündgen R (1981) Subkortikale arteriosklerotische Encephalopathie: klinische, CT-morphologische und elektrophysiologische Befunde. Fortsch Neurol Psychiat 49:223–231
32. Zeumer H, Ringelstein EB, Klose FC (1981) Lakunäre Infarkte im Computertomogramm: Differentialdiagnose, klinische und angiographische Befunde. Fortschr Röntgenstr 134:488–494
33. Zeumer H, Schonsky B, Sturm KW (1980) Predominant white matter involvement in subcortical arteriosclerotic encephalopathy (Binswanger Disease). J Comput Assist Tomogr 4:14–19
34. Zeumer H, Hacke W (1986) Ischämische Insulte. In: Hacke W (ed) Neurologische Intensivmedizin. perimed, Erlangen
35. Zülch KJ (1985) The cerebral infarct. Pathology, pathogenesis and computed tomography. Springer, Berlin Heidelberg New York Tokyo

Part II
Therapeutic Concepts of Stroke Patients

Platelet Inhibitors and the Prevention of Stroke

H. J. KRZYWANEK [1] and H. K. BREDDIN [1]

The Role of Platelets in Atherosclerosis

In recent years increasing evidence has accumulated that platelets play a major role not only in primary hemostasis but also in arterial thrombosis and the progression of the atherosclerotic lesions of the vessel wall. A great variety of laboratory tests have shown enhanced platelet function in patients with vascular disease, e.g., enhanced platelet aggregation, formation of "in vivo aggregates," shortening of platelet life span, and liberation of platelet constituents such as β-TG of PF 4. In the mid 1970s the arachidonic acid pathway was discovered [1], and the theory of a hemostatic balance between thromboxane (TXA_2) and prostacyclin (PGI_2) was postulated. TXA_2 is formed in the platelet and has platelet-aggregating and vasoconstrictive properties. PGI_2 is generated by the endothelial cell of the vessel wall. This substance inhibits platelet aggregation and is a potent vasodilator, thus having antithrombotic properties (Fig. 1).

Acetylsalicylic acid (ASA, aspirin) inhibits both the formation of TXA_2 and PGI_2. The inhibition of TXA_2 is irreversible, lasting for the lifespan of the afflicted platelet population. This means that a single dose of 0.5 g ASA inhibits platelet aggregation for up to 10 days. By contrast, the inhibition of PGI_2 is reversible. Recently a controversy has developed around the question of the optimal dose of ASA which should be used in the prevention of thrombotic complications of atherosclerotic vascular disease. On theoretical grounds, extremely low doses of 30 mg/day [2] or even 40 mg every 2nd day [3] have been proposed, which inhibit TXA_2 production while PGI_2 formation is not affected. By this regimen a strong inhibition of platelet aggregation should be achieved.

The problem is, that at the moment, it is not known which of the many partial functions of the thrombocyte is clinically most important for the progression of atherosclerosis and its complications. It should be clearly pointed out that

(1) inhibition of platelet aggregation is not necessarily accompanied by an antithrombotic effect, and,
(2) the profile of actions that an ideal inhibitor of platelet function should have, has yet to be established.

[1] Department of Internal Medicine, Division of Angiology, J.W. Goethe-University Hospital, Theodor Stern Kai 7, D-6000 Frankfurt/Main 70, FRG

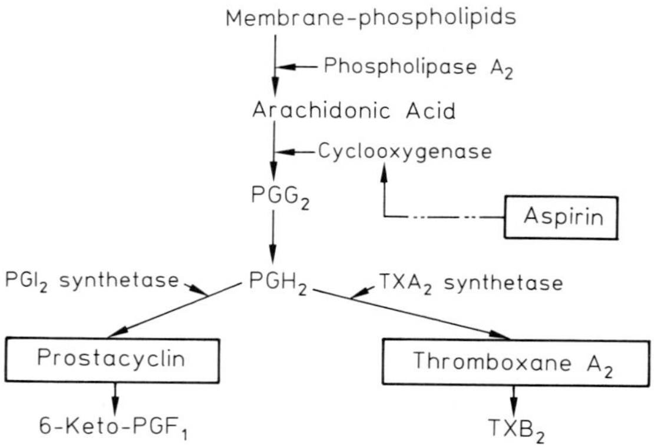

Fig. 1. The arachidonic acid pathway. ASA inhibits the formation of prostacyclin and thromboxane A_2 by inhibiting cyclooxygenase. *Broken line*, inhibition

Inhibitors of Platelet Function

Three platelet function inhibiting drugs have been tested thus far in clinical trials in the prevention of stroke: acetylsalicylic acid (ASA, aspirin), dipyridamole (Persantin) and sulfinpyrazone (Anturano). The modes of action of the three drugs are different (Table 1). ASA is the most potent inhibitor of platelet function in clinical use. It inhibits adhesion and shape change, completely blocks platelet aggregation for the lifespan of the platelet by inhibition of cyclooxygenase and inhibits the release of platelet constituents (PF 3, PF 4, β-TG). The effects of oral administration of a single dose of ASA (250 – 1000 mg) can be measured for

Table 1. Changes in platelet function after single doses of 250 – 100 mg ASA

Short-term effects (4 – 10 h)	Inhibition of adhesion Inhibition of shape change
Medium-term effects (12 – 36 h)	Inhibition of platelet factor 3 availability
Long-term effects (3 – 6 days)	Inhibition of aggregation

Table 2. Effects of platelet-function inhibitors

Mode of action	ASA	Dipyridamole	Sulfinpyrazone
Prolongation of bleeding time	+	–	–
Inhibition of adhesion	+	+	–
Inhibition of shape change	+	+	–
Inhibition of aggregation	+	(+)	+
Prolongation of platelet halflife	–	+	+
Inhibition of cyclooxygenase	+	–	(+)
Inhibition of release of:			
PF 3	+	–	–
PF 4	+	–	+
β-TG	+	+	+

+, strong effect; (+), weak effect; –, no effect

various lengths of time (Table 2). One can differentiate short-term, intermediate-term and long-term effects on platelet function. Sulfinpyrazone and dipyridamole are weak inhibitors of aggregation. In contrast to ASA a prologtion of the shortened platelet half-life can be observed in patients with atherosclerosis.

Clinical Trials with Inhibitors of Platelet Function in Patients with Transient Ischemic Attacks

Nine controlled clinical trials have been published since 1977 on the prevention of stroke in patients with cerebrovascular disease. ASA (1.0 – 1.5 g/day) was used versus placebo, oral anticoagulants and sulfinpyrazone, both as a single medication, and in combination with dipyridamole or sulfinpyrazone. Dipyridamole (225 – 300 mg/day) was administered only in combination with ASA. Sulfinpyrazone was tested in daily doses of 800 mg and in combination with 1.3 g ASA. It is very difficult if not impossible to compare the results of the nine studies, as they differ in the criteria for patient recruitment, end points, observation time and drug combinations. All studies were performed with high-dose ASA. Although one cannot pool the accumulated data for statistical analysis, a trend is demostrable in favour of ASA in the prevention of stroke.

The first double-blind trial of ASA for the treament of patients with cerebral ischemia (AITIA) was published in 1977 by Fields et al. [4]. Here 178 patients with carotid transient ischemic attacks (TIAs) were randomly allocated to 1.3 g ASA/day ($n = 88$) or placebo ($n = 90$). The incidence of subsequent death, cerebral infarction, and retinal infarction were determined as absolute end points. After 27 months of follow-up there was a significant difference in favor of aspirin when the incidence of subsequent TIAs was analyzed (18.3% versus 45.7%). There were fewer absolute end points in the patients under ASA who had carotid artery lesions on the side of their symptoms. At 24 months only those patiens, who had a history of multiple TIAs before recruitment had benefited from ASA treatment considering absolute end points. From the results of this study one can conclude that regular ASA intake is useful in the prevention of recurrent TIAs. It cannot be inferred from the study that ASA prevents stroke, since only the subgroup of patients with a history of multiple TIAs benefited from the treatment.

In another controlled trial [5] 125 patients who had carotid TIAs with subsequent reconstructive operations were randomly allocated to ASA treatment (1.3 g/day; $n = 65$) or placebo ($n = 60$). The follow-up period was 2 years. This revealed a significant difference in favor of ASA if deaths which were not stroke-related were eliminated from the analysis. Considering the recurrence of TIAs in the 6 months following carotid endarterectomy, there was a trend in favor of ASA that did not reach the 5% level of significance. It is interesting to note that eight placebo patients reaching end points within 24 months of observation had brain infarcts. Among patients treated with ASA one cerebral and one retinal infarct occurred and six cardiovascular deaths. The small number of patients and the short period of follow-up do not permit the conclusion that ASA has an effect in preventing stroke.

In the Canadian Cooperative Study [6] 585 patients with at least one cerebral or retinal ischemic attack in the 3 months before entry were followed for an average of 26 months to determine whether ASA (1.3 g/day; $n = 144$), sulfinpyrazone (800 mg/day; $n = 156$), or the combination of the two ($n = 146$) were superior to placebo ($n = 139$) regarding the subsequent occurrence of TIAs, stroke, or death. ASA reduced the risk of stroke of death by 31% ($p < 0.05$). However, this effect was sexdependent: whereas among men the risk reduction for stroke or death was 48% ($p < 0.005$), there was no significant trend observed among women. Sulfinpyrazone did not reduce the incidence of TIAs, and the 10% reduction of stroke or death was not statistically significant. The combination of ASA with sulfinpyrazone had no additional effect on the frequency of cerebrovascular events. The conclusion from the outcome of the Canadian study is that ASA is the drug of choice in the treatment of men at risk of stroke.

Reuther et al. [7] observed 31 patients with carotid TIAs or PRINDs and 27 patients with vertebrobasilar insufficiency for 24 months after randomization to 1.5 g ASA daily or placebo. Five cerebral infarcts occurred during the observation period, four in the placebo group, one 3 weeks after termination of aspirin treatment. The reduction of TIAs in patients taking aspirin was significant, especially in those with a history of multiple attacks ($p < 0.01$). There was no positive trend for aspirin in the patients with vertebrobasilar symptoms.

In the Italian double-blind multicenter study [8] 124 TIA patients with symptoms in the 3 months prior to recruitment were randomly allocated to treatment with ASA (1 g/day; $n = 63$) or sulfinpyrazone (800 mg/day; $n = 61$). Stroke, myocardial infarction, vascular death and recurrence of TIAs were defined as end points. During the observation period of 2 years, 23 events occurred in the ASA group and 25 in the sulfinpyrazone group. In males, a significant benefit in favor of ASA was observed with a 53% risk reduction for further events.

In the French AICLA study [9] 604 patients with cerebral ischemic events, either transient (16%) or complete (84%) and referrable to carotid or vertebrobasilar circulation, were randomized to treatment with ASA (1 g/day; $n = 198$), ASA + dipyridamole (1 g + 225 mg/day; $n = 202$) or placebo ($n = 204$). End points were fatal and nonfatal cerebral infarctions within 3 years of follow-up. At the end of the study the number of end points was 31 in the placebo group, 17 in the ASA group and 18 in the ASA-dipyridamole group, the cumulative incidence being 18% in the placebo group and 10.5% in the two-treatment groups. The conclusion from the outcome of this study is that treatment with ASA has a beneficial effect in the secondary prevention of stroke. The combination of ASA with dipyridamole has no additional effect.

Another clinical trial on the effectiveness of ASA in the prevention of stroke in patients with TIAs was reported by Danish investigators [10]. Here, 203 patients with at least one reversible ischemic attack of less than 72 h duration during the last month prior to admission were randomly assigned to treatment with aspirin (1 g/day; $n = 101$) or placebo ($n = 102$). The average follow-up period was 25 months. No statistically significant differences were found between the treatment groups regarding stroke and death; the incidence was 20.8% in the ASA group and 16.7% in the placebo group. In this trial there was no reduction of recurrent TIAs under ASA treatment. Fewer myocardial infarctions were observed

Table 3. Prospective clinical trials with ASA in cerebral ischemia

Authors	End points	Drug	Dose/day	Drug		Placebo		Follow-up (years)
				n	% End points	*n*	% End points	
Fields et al. (1977)	TIA; death; cerebral, retinal infarct; cardiovasc. death	ASA	1.3 g	88	18.3	90	45.7	0.5
Fields et al. (1978)	cerebral + cardiovasc. death; TIA	ASA	1.3 g	65	11.5	60	24.5	2
Reuther et al. (1980)	TIA; cerebral infarct	ASA	1.5 g	29	20.7	29	44.8	
Barnett et al. (1978)	Total mortality	ASA	1.3 g	144	18.1	139	21.6	2
	TIA; cerebral	Sulf.	800 mg	156	24.4			
	infarct	ASA	1.3 g	146	13.7			
		+ Sulf.	800 mg	146	13.7			
Candelise et al. (1982)	Stroke; TIA;	ASA	1.0 g	63	36.5			2
	vasc. death		800 mg	61	41.0			
Bousser et al. (1983)	fatal, nonfatal	ASA	1.0 g	198	10.5	204	18	3
	stroke	ASA	1.0 g	202	10.5			
		+ Dip.	225 mg					
Sorensen et al. (1983)	stroke; death	ASA	1.0 g	101	20.8	102	16.7	2
Garde et al. (1983)	recurrent TIA;	ASA	1.0 g	127	14.2		1.7	
	fatal, nonfatal stroke	oral A.C.		114	18.4		(20 months)	
Fields et al. (1985)	fatal, nonfatal	ASA	1.3 g	442	14.0			2
	stroke; retinal	ASA	1.3 g	448	12.0			
	infarcts	+ Dip.	300 mg					

Sulf., sulfinpyrazone; Dip., dipyridamole; oral A.C.; oral anticoagulent in the ASA group (5.9%) than in the placebo group (13.7%), but the difference was statistically not significant. This study has received serious criticism concerning the validity of its results [11]. Because of the great number of dropouts only a very small number of patients (77 in the ASA and 71 in the placebo group) remained under observation. A number of risk factors were unequally distributed in the two treatment groups, most of them favoring the placebo group, which might have influenced the outcome of the study.

In a Swedish study [12] 241 patients with symptoms of carotid TIAs (104 with complete recovery, 137 with residual symptoms) were treated either with ASA (1 g/day; $n = 127$) or with oral anticoagulants ($n = 114$). Of the thrombotest values, 77.4% were within, 16.9% above, and 5.7% below the therapeutic range. End points were TIAs with or without residual symptoms, stroke, and death. The observation period was 20 months. Twenty-four end points occurred in the anticoagulant group (18.4%) and 21 in the ASA group (14.2%); the difference is statistically not significant. There were fewer hemorrhages (three versus eight) but more gastrointestinal complaints (five versus none) in the ASA group. Four cerebral infarcts were recorded in each treatment group. The conclusion from the results of this trial is that ASA treatment of patients with TIAs is as effective as anticoagulant therapy but with fewer serious side effects (bleeding complications).

The Persantine Aspirin Trial [13] was conducted in 15 centers in the USA and Canada. The study focussed on the question of whether administration of the combination of ASA and dipyridamole would result in a lower incidence of cerebral of retinal infarction or death than administration of ASA alone for patients with a history of recent carotid TIAs. The 890 patients received either ASA (325 mg) plus placebo or ASA (325 mg) plus dipyridamole (75 mg) four times daily. Of the patients, 98% were followed for at least 1 year, many for 4–5 years. Regarding fatal or nonfatal stroke and retinal infarcts as end points, 60 events occurred in the ASA group and 53 in the ASA-dipyridamole group (not significant). No treatment group difference was found for males versus females or regarding previous TIA history (single of multiple attacks before randomization). The incidence of fatal and nonfatal myocardial infarction and the overall mortality was equal for the two treatment groups. The conclusion from the results of this study is that the patient on ASA therapy for the prevention of recurrent ischemic cerebral attacks gains no further benefit if dipyridamole is administered in addition to ASA.

Conclusion

From the results of the presented clinical studies one can conclude the following:

1. The regular intake of 1.0–1.5 g ASA per day reduces the risk of TIAs in patients with cerebrovascular disease. It is doubtful, whether ASA is of use in the prevention of stroke and cerebrovascular death.
2. Oral anticoagulants are comparably effective, with a higher risk of hemorrhagic complications. Thus, ASA is to be preferred in the treatment of cerebrovascular disease.

3. Dipyridamole and sulfinpyrazone have no additional effect given in combination with ASA; ASA appears the drug of choice.
4. Presently no proof exists that low-dose ASA (50–100 mg/day or less) prevents thrombotic complications or the progression of atherosclerotic vascular disease.

References

1. Moncada S, Vane JR (1979) Arachidonic acid metabolites and the interaction between platelets and blood vessel wall. N Engl J Med 300:1142–1147
2. Patrignani P, Filabozzi P, Patrono C (1982) Selective cumulative inhibition of platelet thromboxane production by low-dose aspirin in healthy subjects. J Clin Invest 69:1366–1372
3. Hanley SP, Beran J, Cockbill SR, Heptinstall S (1982) A regimen for low-dose aspirin. Br Med J 285:1299–1302
4. Fields WS, Lemak NA, Frankowski RF, Hardy RJ (1977) Controlled trial of aspirin in cerebral ischemia. Stroke 8:301–316
5. Fields WS, Lemak NA, Frankowski RF, Hardy RJ (1978) Controlled trial of aspirin in cerebral ischemia. Part II: Surgical group. Stroke 9:309–319
6. The Canadian Cooperative Study Group (1978) A randomized trial of aspirin and sulfinpyrazone in threatened stroke. N Engl J Med 299:53–59
7. Reuther R. Dorndorf W, Loew D (1980) Behandlung transitorisch-ischämischer Attacken mit Acetylsalicylsäure. Münch Med Wochenschr 122:795–798
8. Candelise L, Landi G, Perrone P, Bracchi M, Brambilla G (1982) A randomized trial of aspirin and sulfinpyrazone in patients with TIA. Stroke 13:175–179
9. Bousser MG, Eschwege E, Haguenau M, Lefaucconnier JM, Thibult N, Touboul D, Touboul PJ (1983) "AICLA" controlled trial of aspirin and dipyridamole in the secondary prevention of athero-thrombotix cerebral ischemia. Stroke 14:5–14
10. Sorensen PS, Pedersen H, Marquardsen J, Petersson H, Heltberg A, Simonsen N, Munck O, Andersen LA (1983) Acetylsalicylic acid in the prevention of stroke in patients with reversible cerebral ischemic attacks. A Danish cooperative study. Stroke 14:15–22
11. Dyken ML (1983) Editorial: transient ischemic attacks and aspirin, stroke and death; negative studies and type II error. Stroke 14:2–4
12. Garde A, Samuelsson K, Fahlgren H, Hedberg E, Hjerne LG, Östman J (1983) Treatment after transient ischemic attacks: a comparison between anticoagulant drug and inhibition of platelet aggregation. Stroke 14:677–681
13. The American-Canadian Cooperative Study Group (1985) Persantine aspirin trial in cerebral ischemia. Part II: Endpoint results. Stroke 16:406–415

Anticoagulants in the Treatment of Stroke

J. MARSHALL [1]

Introduction

Before addressing the question of the place of anticoagulant therapy in the treatment of strokes we must first ask what it is that we are endeavouring to treat. Stroke is a clinical syndrome with various pathological causes. Clearly, treating strokes due to cerebral haemorrhage with anticoagulants would be highly inappropriate. Happily this dilemma no longer faces us as it did in the early days of anticoagulant therapy. CT scanning, which is mandatory before embarking on the treatment of stroke, clearly distinguishes between haemorrhage and infarction.

But it is within the realm of infarction itself that there is need to define more clearly what we are treating. When anticoagulants of the phenindione and coumarin type were first introduced, infarction was thought generally to be the result of thrombosis in situ. Embolic infarction was recognised but considered to be responsible in only 5% of cases. The heart was seen as the source of these emboli, the conditions of rheumatic valvular disease with atrial fibrillation, acute myocardial infarction and subacute bacterial endocarditis being commonly held responsible. The studies of Blackwood et al. [2] and Torvik and Jorgensen [10–13] showed this view of infarction to be inaccurate, and demonstrated by autopsy that almost 50% of infarcts are embolic in origin. Stimulated by these observations, a number of stroke surveys, including the Harvard Cooperative Registry and the Framingham Study extending over 4000 stroke patients, have shown that embolism, as diagnosed clinically, is responsible in 6%–23% of cases of stroke. This still falls short of the autopsy figures, but the gap is less than it had previously been.

This gap is in part due to the fact that embolism is only diagnosed clinically when a source can be detected in the heart. There is, however, another important source of emboli, namely atheromatous lesions in the great vessels [8]. Emboli from this source are not usually designated as such clinically, but are labelled as, for example, carotid stenosis or occlusion. Nevertheless, they probably contribute 15%–20% of cerebral emboli. If, in addition, allowance is made for the fact that clinical recognition of emboli cannot be as accurate as recognition at autopsy, the discrepancy between the clinical and pathological surveys is explicable.

Not only has there been a change of view about the frequency of emboli but also about the cardiac conditions responsible. Non-valvular atrial fibrillation

[1] Institute of Neurology, National Hospital for Nervous Diseases, Queen Square, London WC1N 3BG, UK

(NVAF) now heads the list of such conditions and is thought to be responsible for as much as 45% of embolic strokes [7]. Certainly, patients with NVAF show a fivefold increase in the risk of stroke. Other conditions which give rise to emboli are acute myocardial infarction, ventricular aneurysm and prosthetic cardiac valves, in addition to many less frequent causes, such as subacute bacterial endocarditis, mitral valve prolapse, non-rheumatic calcific valvular disease, cardiomyopathy, atrial myxoma, non-bacterial thrombotic endocarditis, and various dysrhythmias.

Mode of Action of Anticoagulants

This new knowledge has an important bearing on our expectations of anticoagulant therapy. Anticoagulants of the coumarin type are most effective against the type of thrombus to be found in veins; this is clot-like, contains substantial fibrin and has a "white tail" of leucocytes. Coumarin prevents the formation and disintegration of the "white tail"; it is not as effective in promoting re-canalisation at the main thrombus itself. Thrombus in the left atrium of the heart is of this type, hence coumarin can be expected to help here.

Thrombus on atheromatous lesions in the great extracranial arteries is not of this type. This contains little fibrin but large aggregations of platelets. Coumarin is not as effective here, and antiplatelet agents may be preferred. Similarly, thrombus in situ in the cerebral arteries is mainly of platelet-aggregation type and is not as responsive to coumarin.

Not only, therefore, must it be recognised that a higher proportion of cerebral infarcts are caused by emboli than was formerly supposed, but the emboli themselves are of different kinds vis-à-vis their responsiveness to coumarin-like drugs.

Empirical Evidence

The theoretical basis for anticoagulant therapy in stroke outlined above cannot be our sole guide in treating patients; we must also consider the empirical evidence regarding its value provided by clinical trials. The obvious starting point is with acute embolism from the heart, as it is here that the case for the use of anticoagulants is strongest. Inevitably the evidence from the literature is conflicting – less concerning whether anticoagulants should be used than when their use should be started.

Prophylaxis of Embolism from the Heart

Preventing acute embolism would be better than preventing recurrence after the first embolism has occurred. The epidemiological evidence quoted above has established a number of risk factors, pre-eminently non-rheumatic or NVAF which shows a fivefold increase in the risk of stroke. There is, therefore, a strong case for prophylactic anticoagulant therapy in this situation. Assessment of its value by controlled clinical trial is urgently required.

Acute Embolism from the Heart

Once infarction has occurred the question of when to start therapy is crucial and controversial. The literature abounds with anecdotal papers describing worsening of embolic infarction following anticoagulants because of haemorrhage into the infarct. For this reason it has been suggested that the initiation of therapy be delayed for 2–3 weeks. This would seem sensible were it not for the risk of recurrence of embolism which various series have shown to occur in 2%–22% of cases within the first 2 weeks (Cerebral Embolism Task Force 1986). Clearly the question is one of balancing risk. There has been only one randomised controlled trial of immediate anticoagulation of embolic stroke reported thus far [6] but as there were only 45 patients, the numbers are insufficient to draw firm conclusions. Only two patients developed haemorrhagic infarction, neither of whom was receiving anticoagulants. Two likewise experienced early recurrent embolism, both also in the non-treated group. There are also in the literature seven non-randomised trials which suggest an appreciable reduction in the recurrence rate, with only one non-randomised trial reporting an opposite result. On balance, therefore, the evidence points to early anticoagulation of embolic infarction being safe, subject to certain provisos. CT scan should not show evidence of haemorrhage in the infarct before anticoagulants are started. Also, early anticoagulation of very large infarcts should be avoided. With these exclusions anticoagulation appears to reduce the risk of recurrent emboli without significant increase of the risk of worsening due to haemorrhage into the infarct.

Stroke in Evolution

The mechanisms underlying stroke in evolution are ill understood and hard to define in the individual case. In some instances increasing neurological deficit is the result of oedema formation which does not call for anticoagulant therapy. In these cases evolution usually follows a period of initial stability. It is in cases in which the deficit slowly increases from the onset that the possibility exists of retrograde spread of arterial thrombosis and occlusion of more branches of the parent artery. Because of the nature of arterial thrombi anticoagulant therapy may not be expected to be effective in this situation. However, two controlled trials [5, 1] have shown trends towards arrest of progression of the deficit and reduced mortality. Whilst the evidence can be controverted, it provides sufficient basis for recommending treatment of the individual case.

Transient Ischaemic Attacks

A transient ischaemic attack (TIA) is a clinical syndrome, not a pathological entity. Nevertheless, the evidence indicates that the majority of TIAs are embolic, most often from atheromatous lesions in the great vessels of the neck. There is, therefore, a prima facie case for considering the use of anticoagulants although coumarin might not be as effective as antiplatelet agents. The empirical evidence on the use of coumarin in a number of trials has been reviewed by Brust [3] who concluded that although the value of anticoagulants in TIAs is unproven, several studies show a trend in their favour. Resolution of this problem is now rendered difficult by the advent of antiplatelet agents and the evidence that they are of benefit in limited groups of patients with TIAs [4]. Comparisons of anticoagulants and antiplatelet agents have been carried out in three trials without any difference being established, although both groups did better than controls. As antiplatelet agents are safer than anticoagulants, they should be the preferred treatment, anticoagulants being reserved for those cases which fail to respond.

Non-embolic Infarction

Infarction following thrombosis of a cerebral artery might not be expected to benefit from coumarin. Unfortunately all relevant trials were carried out before 1965 when CT scanning was not available to distinguish haemorrhage from infarction, and there was little awareness of the need to separate embolic from non-embolic infarction. The trials were on the effect of anticoagulants in completed stroke, a clinical not a pathological entity. In the event they showed no benefit for the treated group [14].

Risk of Haemorrhage

No discussion of anticoagulant therapy is complete without reference to the risk of haemorrhage. The literature on this has recently been reviewed by Levine and Hirsch [9]. Reports of major bleeding episodes range from 2% – 22% of cases per annum and fatal bleedings from 2% – 9%. Hypertension is undoubtedly a risk factor, increasing the risk of bleeding at least twofold. Benefit from anticoagulants needs to be substantial to outweigh this risk; this degree of benefit would only seem to be clearly present in emboli from the heart.

Conclusion

Indications for the use of anticoagulants of the coumarin type in stroke remain unsatisfactory. There is, however, broad agreement between what might be expected from experimental work on their mode of action and the results of clinical trials. There is good indication for anticoagulants in the prevention and treatment of cerebral infarcts caused by cardiac emboli. Their role in TIAs is less certain; antiplatelet agents are the agent of choice. There is no place for anticoagulants in non-embolic cerebral infarction.

References

1. Baker RN, Broward JA, Fang HC, Fisher CM, Groch SN, Heyman A, Karp HR, McDevitt E, Scheinberg P, Schwartz W, Toole JF (1962) Anticoagulant therapy in cerebral infarction. Report on co-operative study. Neurology 12:823–835
2. Blackwood W, Hallpike JF, Kocen RS, Mair WGP (1969) Atheromatous disease of the carotid arterial system and embolism from the heart in cerebral infarction: a morbid anatomical study. Brain 92:897–910
3. Brust JCM (1977) Transient ischemic attacks: natural history and anticoagulation. Neurology 27:701–707
4. Canadian Cooperative Study Group (1978) A randomized trial of aspirin and sulfinpyrazone in threatened stroke. N Engl J Med 299:53–59
5. Carter AB (1961) Anticoagulant treatment in progressing stroke. Br Med J 2:70–73
6. Cerebral Embolism Study Group (1983) Immediate anticoagulation of embolic stroke. A randomised trial. Stroke 14:668–674
7. Cerebral Embolism Task Force (1986) Cardiogenic brain embolism. Arch Neurol 43:71–84
8. Gunning AJ, Pickering GW, Robb-Smith AHT, Ross Russell R (1964) Mural thrombosis of the internal carotid artery and subsequent embolism. Q J Med 33:155–195
9. Levine M, Hirsh J (1986) Hemorrhagic complications of long-term anticoagulant therapy for ischemic cerebral vascular disease. Stroke 17:111–116
10. Torvik A, Jorgensen L (1964) Thrombotic and embolic occlusions of the carotid arteries in an autopsy material. Part 1. Prevalence, location and associated diseases. J Neurol Sci 1:24–39
11. Torvik A, Jorgensen L (1966) Thrombotic and embolic occlusions of the carotid arteries in an autopsy series. Part 2. Cerebral lesions and clinical course. J Neurol Sci 3:410–432
12. Jorgensen L, Torvik A (1966) Ischaemic cerebrovascular diseases in an autopsy series. Part 1. Prevalence, location and predisposing factors in verified thromboembolic occlusions, and their significance in the pathogenesis of cerebral infarction. J Neurol Sci 3:490–509
13. Jorgensen L, Torvik A (1969) Ischaemic cerebrovascular diseases in an autopsy series. Part 2. Prevalence, location, pathogenesis, and clinical course of cerebral infarcts. J Neurol Sci 9:285–320
14. Weksler BB, Lewin M (1983) Anticoagulation in cerebral ischemia. Stroke 14:658–663

Risk and Benefit of Anticoagulation in Patients with Acute Hemispheric Infarctions: Preliminary Results of a Prospective Study

G. KORBMACHER[1] and E. B. RINGELSTEIN[1]

Introduction

In clinical practice neurologists are often confronted with stroke patients who are at high risk of recurrent stroke. Approximately 12% of patients who have had cardiogenic brain embolism experience reinfarction within a 2-week period after the initial attack [4–6, 14] (Table 1). This rate is similar to that for most cardiac sources of emboli (Table 2) except for nonvalvular atrial fibrillation, which seems to be characterized by a lower risk of reinfarction [4–6, 22]. This does not contradict the fact that nonvalvular atrial fibrillation is the most frequent source of cerebral embolism [6, 22, 24, 27], particularly at the time of onset of dysrhythmia [17].

Apart from the prevention of cardiac embolism, anticoagulation with heparin and/or coumarin is thought to be beneficial for patients with dissecting aneurysms [11] and for those with high-grade symptomatic stenoses of the internal carotid artery (ICA), if endarterectomy is not immediately possible (e.g., "pseudo-occlusion", [19]). It does not, however, appear to be effective in cases of so-called progressive lacunes [7]. Anticoagulation is also recommended in particular types of inflammatory angiopathies [15]. Arteriosclerotic intracranial large vessel stenoses are not generally accepted as an indication for anticoagulant therapy (see Mashall, this volume). However, in our experience heparin and/or coumarin therapy in high-grade stenoses of the middle cerebral or vertebrobasilar arteries leads to prompt cessation of transient ischemic attacks and prevents progression of neurological deficits. Controlled prospective studies since the advent of CT scanning are still lacking. This list of various cardiac and cerebrovascular disorders underlines the clinical importance of anticoagulation as a major therapeutic approach in a broad spectrum of stroke etiologies.

The *risk of cerebral hemorrhage* makes clinicians hesitate in advocating early anticoagulation in patients with recent brain infarctions. In the literature, reports of this risk range from 0% to 24% (Table 3) [5, 6, 18]. Unfortunately, this risk has only been evaluated in retrospective studies or in small cohorts. The present study was performed prospectively in order better to define the risk of brain hemorrhage during anticoagulation with heparin and to demonstrate its clinical benefit as assessed by the reinfarction rate.

---

[1] Department of Neurology, Klinikum RWTH, University Hospital, D-5100 Aachen, FRG

Table 1. Studies on the probability of recurrence of brain infarction in stroke patients suffering from embolizing heart disease. (According to Cerebral Embolism Task Force 1986)

Author	Reference	Cardiac source of emboli	*n*	Observation interval	Percentage recurrent brain embolism
CESG (1983)	[4]	Mixed	20	14 days	10%
Furlan et al. (1982)	[9]	Mixed	23	7 days	22%
Koller (1982)	[13]	Mixed	29	14 days	14%
Sage and van Uitert (1983)	[21]	Atrial fibrillation	59	14 days	2%
Bass (1983)	[1]	Mixed	30	30 days	10%

Table 2. Risk of early recurrent brain embolism after embolic stroke in various heart diseases. (According to Cerebral Embolism Study Group 1983)

Type of heart disease	Observation interval	Mean percentage recurrent brain embolism
Nonvalvular atrial fibrillation	14 days	10%
Rheumatic heart disease	14 days	13%
Acute myocardial infarction	14 days	13%

Methods and Patients

Forty patients (26 males, 14 females) entered the study; their ages ranged from 14 to 77 years (mean, 51.4). All patients had experienced ischemic strokes with visible infarctions on CT. Not admitted were patients with strokes due to cerebral microangiopathies, i.e., with lacunar infarctions or with the typical features of subcortical arteriosclerotic encephalopathy (Binswanger's type) [29, 30]. Patients were also excluded who had had brainstem or cerebellar infarctions, because of the poor quality of CT images in the infratentorial region. And finally, patients with compact hemorrhages were excluded from the study, although those with hemorrhagic infarctions were not. All patients were treated with heparin within 72 h (most within 24 h) after the onset of acute stroke symptoms. The dosage was at least 24000 IU/day and was controlled by PTT (partial thromboplastin time) values, so that PTT increased to 1.5–2.0 times normal (i.e. $1.5-2.0\times 30-45$ s). After a period of at least 2 weeks with heparin the treatment regimen changed to either subsequent coumarin application or antiplatelet agents. In four patients an initial local treatment with 200000 IU urokinase within 2 h was given before administering heparin.

The examination protocol included (a) a daily recheck of the clinical state of the patients in order to detect any deterioration for whatever reason, particularly signs of reinfarction or bleeding; (b) repeated CT scans were performed for each patient not only after at least a 1-week period of heparin treatment but also immediately in any case which presented signs of clinical worsening and/or head-

Table 3. Studies on the risk of cerebral hemorrhage due to early anticoagulation

Author(s)	Reference	*n*	Start of anticoagulent after onset of stroke (h)	Percentage of patients with elevated blood pressure (%)	Percentage of large infarctions (%)	Percentage of visualized symptomatic brain hemorrhage (%)
CESG (1983)	[4]	35	30	23	20	0
Lodder and Van der Lugt (1983)	[14]	21	<24	–	38	0
Furlan et al. (1982)	[9]	25	<24	–	–	0
Koller (1982)	[13]	15	<48	–	–	0
Hart et al. (1983)	[10]	7	28	14	0	0
Shields et al. (1984)	[23]	28	?	–	–	14
Bass (1983)	[1]	71	?	–	–	14
Calendre et al. (1983)	[3]	17	<24	–	–	24

Cerebral Embolism Study Group (1984)

Table 4. Features of hemorrhagic infarction versus frank hemorrhage

Hemorrhagic infarction:
Strictly territorial
Petechial hemorrhage
Mixed areas of low and high density
Frank hemorrhage
Nonterritorial
Compact/confluent clot of blood
Homogeneous density
Often with mass effect

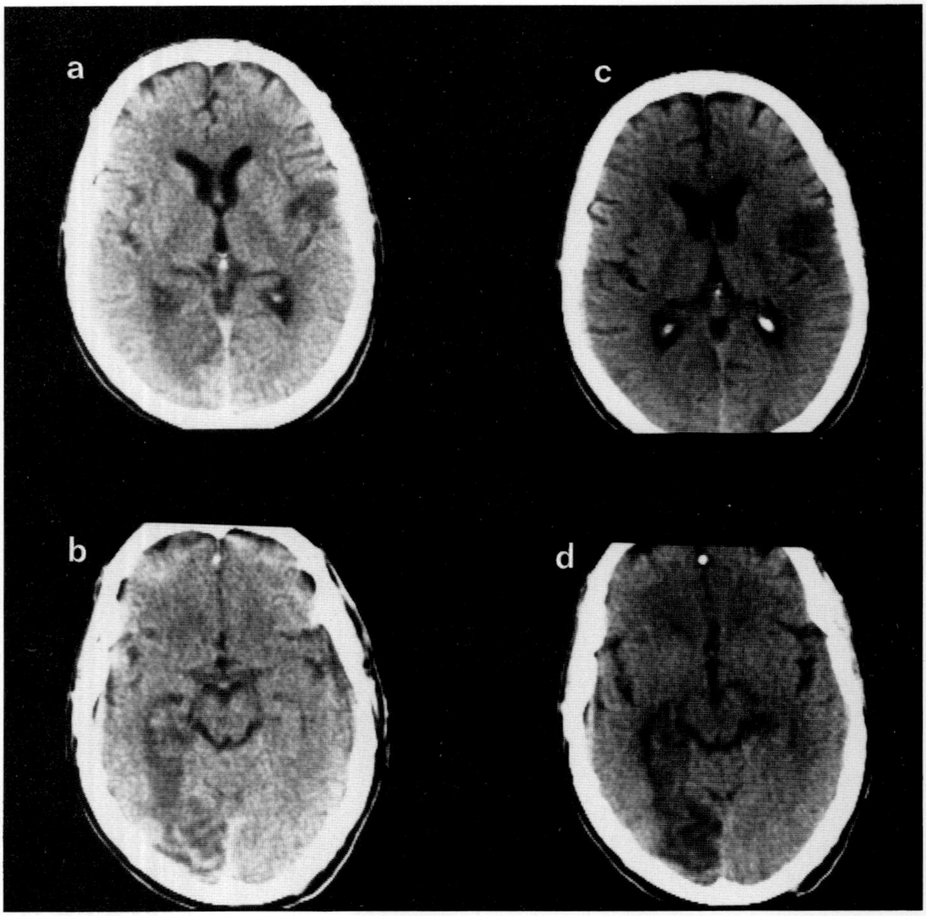

Fig. 1a–d. CT images of a patient with two embolic infarctions, one of them with initial spontaneous hemorrhagic transformation.
a, b Before heparin therapy and within twenty-four hours after acute onset of stroke, both a hypodense territorial infarction within the left MCA territory, and a hemorrhagic infarction of the right posterior cerebral artery territory became visible. **c, d** During the course of heparinization, the hemorrhagic transformation of the PCA infarction disappeared

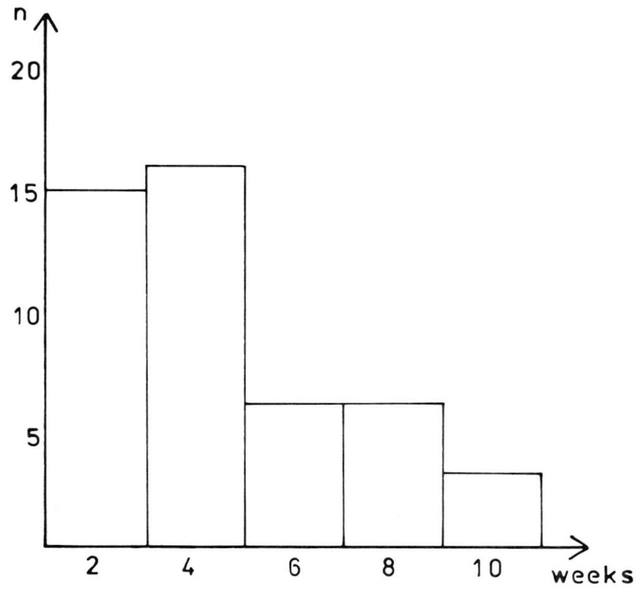

Fig. 2. Duration of heparin treatment. *Abscissa* indicates the duration of heparinization in weeks; *n*, number of patients

ache; (c) patients with visible hemorrhagic transformation of their infarction were reexamined by means of CT over shorter intervals, so that in some patients a series of four or five CT scans were performed.

The criteria for hemorrhagic infarction versus frank hemorrhage are given in Table 4. One of the chief features is the territorial versus non-territorial distribution of the hyperdense lesion. Another quite characteristic criterion for the differentiation of these lesions was the petechial versus compact and confluent type of hemorrhage. As a rule, open hemorrhages presented with compact bleedings and had an immediate severe mass effect. By contrast, hemorrhagic infarctions showed a patchy distribution of hyperdense and hypodense areas.

Results

Forty-four hemispheric infarctions of 40 patients were visualized and were differentiated according to a previously published classification scheme [19, 20] (see also Zeumer and Ringelstein, this volume). This system aims at a pathogenetically oriented classification of ischemic brain lesions principally differentiating between thromboembolic territorial infarctions and hemodynamically induced, nonterritorial lesions. The classification of lesions of this cohort is summarized in Table 5.

An overview of the infarctions under study is shown in Fig. 3, each slice representing one patient. The cut with the largest extension of infarction(s) was chosen as representative. Most of the infarctions were large in size, with diameters of more than 3 cm (Table 6). Heparin was administered only if one of the above

Table 5. Distribution of infarctions by location ($n = 44$)

Location	Number
Territorial infarctions	
Predominantly cortical	33
MCA territory	24
PCA territory	8
ACA territory	1
Purely subcortical	
large ganglionic infarctions	8
Nonterritorial infarctions	
terminal zone infarctions	3

indications was present, or was at least highly suggestive. A list of reasons for anticoagulation treatment in our patients is given in Table 7. In most cases the reason for heparin therapy was cardiac embolism. Underlying heart diseases were quite variable (Table 8) and did not only include nonvalvular atrial fibrillation as in some other studies [10, 21], but a considerable number of cases of ($n = 8$) valvular disease.

Forty-three of 44 infarction were nonhemorrhagic on CT when heparin therapy was started. In one patient was one of two brain infarctions initially slightly hemorrhagic. This lesion was in the territory of the posterior cerebral artery (Fig. 1b). During heparin therapy, however, the hemorrhagic transformation of this infarction vanished, i.e., it was no longer visible in the repeat-CT scan (Fig. 1d). Surprisingly, the infarction of the left MCA territory of this patient did not become hemorrhagic at any time (Fig. 1a, c).

Three out of four patients treated initially with urokinase revealed hemorrhagic transformation of their infarctions during the first 24h. This was not paralleled by clinical deterioration, and patients' deficits remained stable. Despite hemorrhagic transformation of the infarctions, heparin therapy was initiated immediately after the 2-h period of fibrinolysis. Repeated CT scans proved that heparin did not further increase the hemorrhagic component of these infarctions. This was also true for the one case with spontaneous initial hemorrhagic transformation of the infarcted brain area. Quite unexpectedly, the hemorrhagic component resolved gradually during heparin therapy and was no longer visible on repeated CT scans.

Thirty-five of the 43 initially nonhemorrhagic infarctions remained hypodense on repeated CT scan, i.e., did not undergo hemorrhagic transformation during heparin therapy. Five lesions became hyperdense and showed the typical features of hemorrhagic infarctions as described above (Table 4). None of these, however, experienced any clinical worsening, i.e., the hemorrhagic transformations remained clinically silent. These findings are summarized in the flow chart in Fig. 4.

In only one case in which the initial CT revealed minimal petechial hemorrhages within the infarcted area did the subsequent continuation of anticoagulation with *coumarin* lead after a 2-week period of heparin treatment to a confluent bleeding and acute severe headache (but without further neurological deficits).

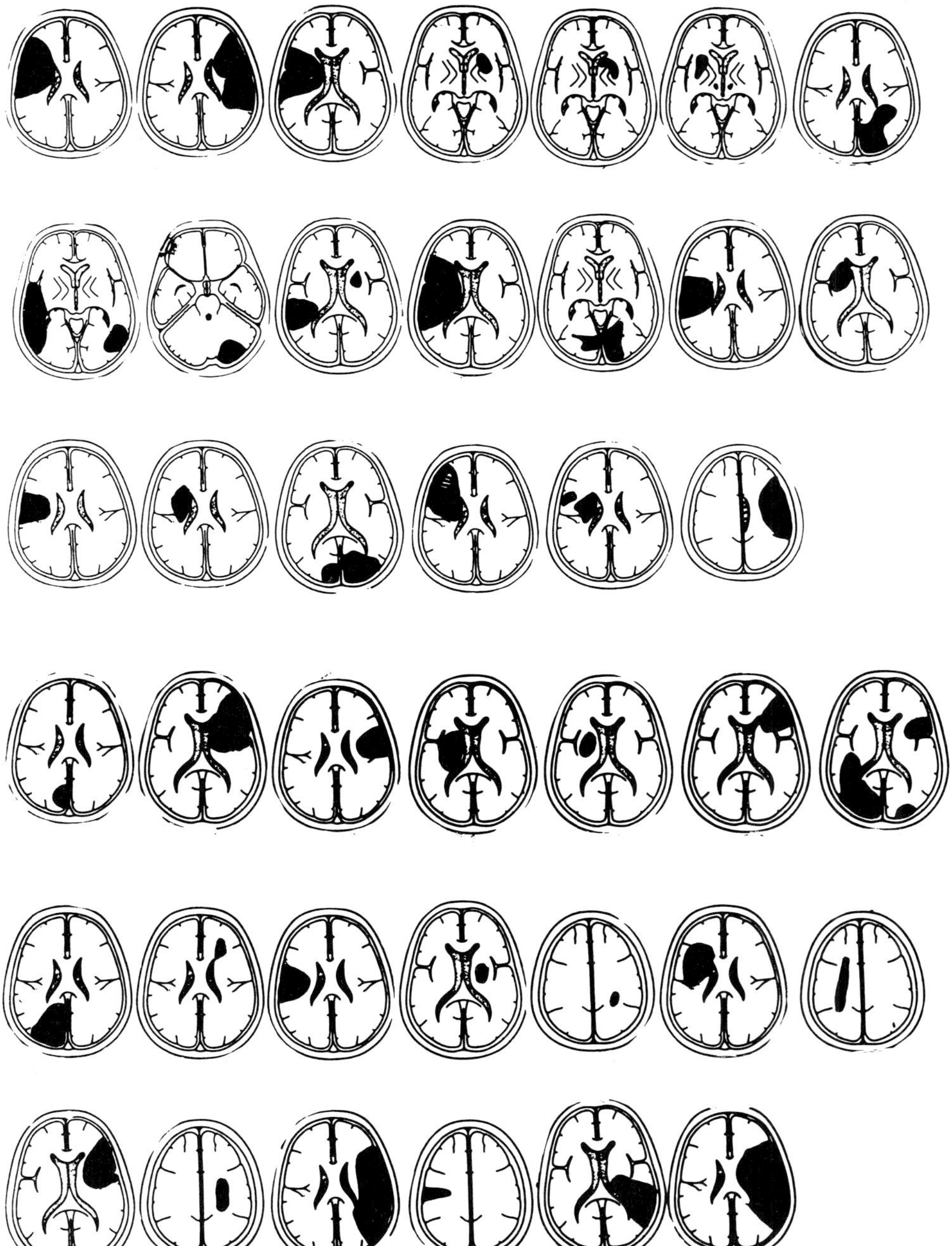

Fig. 3. Size and pattern of the infarcted brain areas of 40 patients. The infarction(s) of each patient is schematically demonstrated in one CT slice with the largest extension of the infarcted tissue. Lesions occurred within the MCA, PCA and ACA territory. The vast majority of infarctions were of territorial and cortical types; hemodynamically induced lesions were rare. The figure also indicates that most of the infarctions were of large size

Table 6. Distribution of infarctions by size ($n = 40$)

Classification	Diameter	Number
Small	≤ 1 cm	1
Medium	1 – 3 cm (e.g., small cortical infarctions or ganglionic infarctions)	17
Large	>3 cm (mostly territorial infarctions of main cerebral arteries)	22

Table 7. Indications for heparin therapy

Indication	*n*
Cardioembolic etiology highly suggestive	22
Intracranial stenosis	6
Extracranial, high-grade stenosis	1
Dissection of the internal carotid artery	2
Vasculitis presumed	2
Paradoxical embolism	1
Catheter-related embolism	1
Stroke due to AT III deficieny	1
Others	4

Table 8. Cardioembolic etiologies ($n = 22$)

Etiology	*n*
Severe cardiac arrhythmia	8
AF	4
PVCs	3
AV block III	1
Left ventricle hypokinesia	3
Left ventricle aneurysm	1
Mitral valve prosthesis	2
Mitral valve stenosis	2
Mitral valve prolaps	4
Nonhypertrophic cardiomyopathy	1
Paradoxical embolism	1

This bleeding occurred accidentally after 6 months because the patient had mistakenly received both antiplatelet agents and coumarin.

No patient suffered a further stroke during heparin therapy, i.e., during a follow-up period of at least 4 weeks.

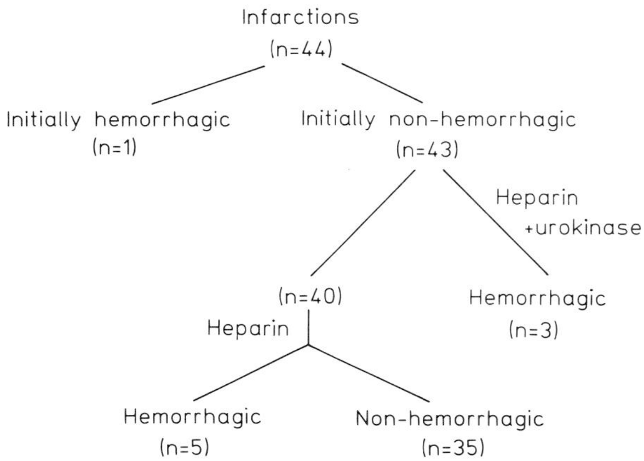

Fig. 4. Flow chart summarizing treatment and CT findings in 44 brain infarctions

Discussion

Although the present study is of a preliminary character, it clearly indicates that heparin therapy of recent brain infarctions is feasible without major risk to the patient. None of the 40 patients revealed any clinical deterioration during the period of treatment. This is also true for the one patient with brain hemorrhage; this occurred later during coumarin therapy in combination with antiplatelet agents. The simultaneous application of any anticoagulative drug with platelet inhibitors is known to entail a high risk of bleeding complications and is considered obsolete [26, 28]. This study, however, was not designed to clarify the risk of brain hemorrhage due to coumarin, but was restricted to the issue of benefits and hazards due to early short-term heparin therapy.

A prospective study such as the present one relies on two prerequisites. The arterial blood pressure must be carefully observed in each patient, the majority of whom here were hypertensive. This is of utmost importance, as has already been outlined in the literature [5]. To our knowledge, however, systemic prospective studies on this problem do not exist yet. The second important aspect is the careful check of coagulation parameters, particularly the partial prothrombin time and antithrombin III activity [25]. This is necessary in order to control the dosage of heparin and to guarantee effectiveness of treatment. As much as a twofold prolongation of the partial prothrombin time is generally thought to indicate an optimal effect of anticoagulation with heparin [4, 16, 25].

Unlike other studies reported in the literature [9, 12, 14], the initial (spontaneous or induced) hemorrhagic transformation of an acute brain infarction was not an exclusion criterion for heparin application in our patients. This unconventional strategy seemed to be justified for several reasons. (a) Previous experience with patients suffering from parenchymatous bleeding of the brain due to sinus thrombosis has indicated that heparin treatment was tolerated without any hazards, particularly without further brain hemorrhages. This favorable finding has recently been confirmed in a retrospective study of patients with cerebral venous thrombosis [2]. (b) Patients with spontaneous hemorrhagic transformation of their infarctions did not reveal further progression of symptoms which could have been attributed to these morphological changes. (c) In another study, only three out of 28 patients with hemorrhagic transformation presented with clinical deterioration, which, however, clearly occurred due to open bleeding [12]. Our findings indicate that hemorrhagic transformation of an ischemic brain infarction obviously does not worsen the patient's state, provided that the hemorrhage is not a frank bleeding.

More frequent CT reexamination presumably would have provided deeper insight into the true time course of the hemorrhagic transformation, thus allowing a better analysis of the causal relationship between these morphological changes and the application of the drug. In our series, the proportion of patients with hemorrhagic transformation was lower than that recently reported in a prospective study with a higher frequency of CT reexamination [12]. It cannot be ruled out that a few hemorrhagic transformations have remained undetected. A more precise CT analysis and follow-up, however, would not have provided additional clinically relevant data for our findings.

The present research design did not allow clarification as to whether early heparin therapy of stroke patients really improves the final outcome. If this had been intended, a randomized study would have been necessary. Nevertheless, none of our patients experienced any reinfarction, although the majority of them were at high risk of acquiring recurrent strokes due to cardiac embolism. We conclude that anticoagulant therapy is very likely to be effective in reducing the recurrence of cardiac embolism, and that it should be employed [8]. Despite these positive findings, heparin therapy remains a distinct and sophisticated type of treatment which requires an indication cautiously based on the pathogenesis of the stroke.

Acknowledgements. The authors are greatly indebted to Professor H. Zeumer and Drs. H. Brückmann, and M. Hutschenreuter for the performance of the CT scans. The careful preparation of the manuscript by Mrs. Kati Seidel is thankfully acknowledged.

References

1. Bass E (1983) Anticoagulation in cerebral embolism. Can J Neurol Sci 10:32–36
2. Bousser MG, Chiras J, Bories J, Castaigne P (1985) Cerebral venous thrombosis – a review of 38 cases. Stroke 16:199–213
3. Calandre L, Ortega JF, Barbejo F, Postera A (1983) Cerebral embolism and anticoagulation (Letter to the Editor). Neurology 33:1103–1104
4. Cerebral Embolism Study Group (1983) Immediate anticoagulation of embolic stroke: a randomized trial. Stroke 14:668–676
5. Cerebral Embolism Study Group (1984) Immediate anticoagulation of embolic stroke: brain hemorrhage and management options. Stroke 15:779–789
6. Cerebral Embolism Task Force (1986) Cardiogenic brain embolism. Arch Neurol 43:71–84
7. Dobkin PH (1983) Heparin for lacunar stroke in progression. Stroke 14:421–423
8. Dyken ML (1983) Anticoagulant and platelet-antiaggregating therapy in stroke and treatened stroke. In: Barnett HJM (ed) Neurologic clinics: cerebrovascular disease. Saunders, Philadelphia, pp 223–242
9. Furlan AJ, Carabier SJ, Hobbs RE (1982) Hemorrhage and anticoagulation after nonseptic embolic brain infarction. Neurology 32:280–282

10. Hart RG, Coull BM, Hart PD (1983) Early recurrent embolism associated with nonvascular atrial fibrillation. Stroke 16:688–693
11. Hart RG, Easton JD (1985) Dissections. Stroke 1:925–927
12. Hornig CR, Dorndorf W, Agnoli AL (1986) Hemorrhagic cerebral infarction – a prospective study. Stroke 17:179–185
13. Koller RL (1982) Recurrent embolic cerebral infarction and anticoagulation. Neurology 32:283–285
14. Lodder J, Van der Lugt PJM (1983) Evaluation of the risk of immediate anticoagulant treatment in patients with embolic stroke of cardiac origin. Stroke 14:42–46
15. Mumenthaler M (1984) Inflammatory angiopathy. In: Toole JF (ed) Cerebrovascular disorders, 3rd edn. Raven, New York, pp 299–312
16. Ott BR, Zamani A, Kleefield J, Funkenstein HH (1986) The clinical spectrum of hemorrhagic infarction. Stroke 17:630–637
17. Petersen P, Godtfredsen J (1986) Embolic complications in paroxysmal atrial fibrillation. Stroke 17:622–626
18. Ramirez-Lassepas M, Quinones MR, Nino HH (1986) Treatment of acute ischemic stroke. Arch Neurol 43:386–390
19. Ringelstein EB, Berg-Dammer E, Zeumer H (1983) The so-called atheromatous pseudoocclusion of the internal carotid artery: a diagnostic and therapeutical challenge. Neuroradiology 25:147–155
20. Ringelstein EB, Zeumer H, Schneider R (1985) Der Beitrag der zerebralen Computertomographie zur Differentialtypologie und Differentialtherapie des ischämischen Großhirninfarktes. Fortschr Neurol Psychiat 9:315–354
21. Sage JS, Van Uitert RL (1983) Risk of recurrent stroke with atrial fibrillation differences between rheumatic and arteriosclerotic heart disease. Stroke 14:537–540
22. Sherman DG, Hart RG, Easton DJ (1986) The secondary prevention of stroke in patients with atrial fibrillation. Arch Neurol 43:68–70
23. Shields RW Jr, Laureno R, Lachman T, Victor M (1984) Anticoagulant-induced hemorrhage in acute cerebral embolism. Stroke 15:426–437
24. Starkey I, Warlow C (1986) The secondary prevention of stroke in patients with atrial fibrillation. Arch Neurol 43:66–67
25. Thompson AR, Harker LA (1983) Manual of hemostasis and thrombosis, 3rd edn. Davis, Philadelphia
26. Torosian M, Michelson EL, Mortganroth J et al. (1978) Aspirin and coumadin-related bleeding after coronary-artery bypass graft surgery. Ann Int Med 89:325–328
27. Wolf PA, Kannel WB, McGee DL, Meeks SL, Bharucha NE, McNamara PM (1983) Duration of atrial fibrillation and imminence of stroke: the framingham study. Stroke 14:664–667
28. Yett HS, Stillmann JJ, Salzman EW (1978) The hazards of heparin plus aspirin. N Engl J Med 298:1092
29. Zeumer H, Schonsky B, Sturm HW (1980) Predominant white matter involvement in subcortical arteriosclerotic encephalopathy (Binswanger disease). J Comput Assist Tomogr 4:14–19
30. Zeumer H, Ringelstein EB, Klose KC (1981) Lakunäre Infarkte im Computertomogramm. Angiographische Befunde und differentialdiagnostische Gesichtspunkte. Fortschr Röntgenstr 4:188–194

tPA and scuPA: New Concepts in the Treatment of Acute Stroke*

G. J. DEL ZOPPO [1]

Introduction

Recombinant DNA techniques have allowed the synthesis of two relatively thrombus-specific thrombolytic enzymes, tissue plasminogen activator (tPA) and single-chain urokinase plasminogen activator (scuPA, pro-urokinase), in quantities sufficient for clinical studies. The possible use of these interesting proteins in the treatment of acute thromboembolic stroke is the subject of this review. The hypothesis that is central to the possible use of these agents is that neurological function may be preserved and ischemic injury reduced if agents which produce dissolution of thrombi are given early in the course of acute thrombotic stroke [1]. Recent experience with local infusion of the conventional thrombolytic agents urokinase and streptokinase imply that fibrin-specific agents may have value in the treatment of acute stroke. The theoretical basis for the use of these agents follows directly from the molecular mechanisms of endogenous thrombolysis.

The Thrombolytic System of Control of Thrombus Growth

Thrombolytic enzymes may be derived from endogenous sources (urokinase, scu PA, tPA) or exogenous sources (streptokinase) and have been developed to effect dissolution of thrombi in pathological conditions [2–7]. Use of thrombolytic agents represents a manipulation of the natural system of thrombus control. This system is promoted by platelet-mediated activation of the coagulation system, as well as activation of the intrinsic system of coagulation [8]. The ultimate effect of activation of the coagulation system is the generation of the serine protease thrombin, which converts fibrinogen to fibrin, and the products of fibrinogen degradation [9, 10]. The formation of a fibrin network for stabilization of the growing thrombus is the result of thrombin-mediated fibrin generation [11].

Several endogenous mechanisms stimulate the conversion of another serine protease, plasminogen, to the active enzyme plasmin which is capable of non-selective degradation of fibrinogen and fibrin [11]. Agents which stimulate

* This work was supported in part by Grant No. Hl31950 od the NIH and Grant No. Ag-2/75-1 of the Deutsche Forschungsgemeinschaft
* This is publication 4650BCR from the Research Institute of Scripps Clinic, La Jolla, California

[1] Department of Basic and Clinical Research, Scripps Clinic and Research Foundation, 10666 North Torrey Pines Road, La Jolla, CA 92037, USA

plasminogen conversion to plasmin serve the function of thrombolytic (fibrinolytic) agents. Therefore, thrombolytic agents are substances which dissolve thrombi by enzymatically cleaving the fibrin framework of the thrombus. Of the endogenous fibrinolytic agents, urokinase nonspecifically activates plasminogen to effect fibrin(ogen) dissolution, while tPA and scuPA appear to activate plasminogen only in the presence of fibrin [2, 7]. Both mechanisms are responsible for in vivo thrombus lysis and undoubtedly contribute to the spontaneous dissolution of arterial thrombotic occlusions observed in patients. The development of the endogenous fibrinolytic agents in quantities sufficient for pharmacological use has been based on the premise that augmentation of the fibrinolytic process by infusion of such agents can lead to timely dissolution of occluding thrombi.

Fibrinolysis and Acute Thrombotic Disease

The conventional thrombolytic agents, urokinase and streptokinase, have been used with relative success in several acute thrombotic disorders. The UPET and USPET studies demonstrated the equal efficacy of urokinase and streptokinase in the treatment of acute pulmonary embolism with cardiovascular instability [12, 13]. Local (intraarterial) infusion of either agent has produced recanalization in patients with acute peripheral arterial occlusion [14–23] and with occlusion of arteriovenous grafts/shunts. In the former, reinstitution of blood flow and recanalization could be expected in 20%–40% of patients, particularly among those with adequate arterial "run-off." Direct intrathrombus infusion of the thrombolytic agents was found to be necessary to produce recanalization [14, 16]. Reperfusion of thrombosed central venous catheters can also be achieved with local infusion of fibrinolytic agents. Recently an extensive experience with intracoronary and intravenous infusion of conventional agents in documented thrombosed coronary arteries of patients presenting with an acute myocardial infarction has led to recanalization rates of 60%–70% [24–42]. It remains debatable whether reinstitution of flow in this setting can lead to improved mortality. The use of fibrinolytic agents, both systemically and locally, in patients with acute venous occlusions has met with less success [43–61]. Although individual patients may derive benefit from this approach, variables important to such success remain unclear.

Unresolved Problems

Although consistent efforts to coordinate and control studies of intravenous and intraarterial infusion of thrombolytic agents in acute coronary artery thrombosis have been made, the optimal treatment regimes for given thrombotic conditions have remained elusive in most cases. This is as much due to the nature, variability and extent, and clinical severity of a given thrombotic disease as to the difficulties involved with assaying the outcome events in a given study. For instance, current clinical assay systems, e.g., tissue metabolic function as indicated by clinical recovery, are often general and crude, while the kinetics of a specific agent, e. g., urokinase/streptokinase, make dose-rate adjustments during therapy difficult. This is particularly true of streptokinase, which does not behave according to first-order kinetics [2, 4]. Plasminogen and fibrinogen depletion are poor indicators of clinical efficacy.

Finally, of major significance is the potential problem of local or distant hemorrhage associated with infusion of the thrombolytic agent. Urokinase and streptokinase, have an apparent two-phase behavior. The initial *fibrinolytic* phase is intrinsic to the activity of each protein. Both proteins also have in common an apparent *anticoagulant* phase, secondary to the inactivation of factors V and VIII, in addition to fibrin(ogen) degradation [2–4]. In contrast, tPA and scuPA do not inactivate factors V and VIII so that the risk of hemorrhage associated with the anticoagulant state is presumably thereby reduced [7, 62, 63]. Recent work indicates a potentiation of the thrombolytic and hemorrhagic properties associated with at least one preparation of tPA when heparin is infused concomitantly [64].

The problem of hemorrhage is compounded by the difficulty of assessing the intrinsic hemorrhagic risk of a given patient. Hemorrhage, as in the case of intracerebral hemorrhage, may result from lysis of thrombi protecting sites of arterial damage; this risk may be increased by the anticoagulant phase when urokinase/streptokinase or the combination of heparin and tPA is used. At the present time, experience with scuPA is inadequate to give a reasonable assessment of the risk of this problem. Theoretically, agents such as tPA and scuPA should be expected to have a lower hemorrhagic potential than urokinase and streptokinase, although in a given patient, this is impossible to assess.

Cerebrovascular Thrombosis

Cerebral angiographic studies within 12 h of the onset of symptoms of acute stroke have demonstrated thrombotic and stenotic lesions in cerebral vessels in the territory appropriate to the symptoms in 70%–80% of patients [65]. This incidence is independent of the vascular territory examined (e.g., carotid territory vs. vertebrobasilar territory). Demonstration of the thrombotic and thromboembolic basis of acute cerebrovascular stroke, and the success of intracoronary thrombolysis during acute myocardial infarction from the basis for the current interest in the use of thrombolytic agents in the treatment of acute stroke. With the advent of relatively fibrin-selective agents, such as tPA and scuPA, the possibility of a local thrombus-directed effect from intravenous infusion becomes theoretically attractive.

Thrombolysis in Cerebrovascular Thrombosis

Early, mostly uncontrolled studies of intravenous thrombolytic agents in (nonacute) stroke patients were interpreted to indicate that thrombolysis does not alter the clinical course of stroke patients, and indeed, could be harmful due to an apparent increased incidence of intracerebral hemorrhage [1, 66–71]. The absence of current radiological diagnostic techniques to rule out hemorrhage as a presenting cause of stroke, inadequate control of the fibrinolytic agents, and late treatment of most patients are evident weaknesses of those studies. More recent experience with intraarterial (local) infusion of urokinase/streptokinase in acute stroke patients with angiographically documented thrombotic occlusions has resulted in thrombus lysis, recanalization in the affected arterial territory, and an incidence of cerebral hemorrhage which is within reported spontaneous hemorrhage rates [1, 72–79]. Individual case reports, joint work at the RWTH in Aachen and at SCRF in La Jolla on middle cerebral artery patients, and a series of 43 vertebrobasilar occlusion patients treated at the RWTH support the conclusion that local thrombolysis can achieve recanalization [1, 80]. Whether this approach can improve morbidity and mortality of territory-specific stroke has not been studied. The ability to achieve local thrombus lysis with interventional neuroradiological techniques limits the availability of this approach to centers with interventional neuroradiological expertise. Therefore, the possible availability of agents which are thrombus-selective may obviate the requirement for invasive delivery of thrombolytic agents in further studies of acute stroke management.

It should be noted that successful arterial recanalization has occurred in patients who were treated within 6–8 h of the onset of symptoms of acute stroke. It is assumed that the risk of hemorrhagic complications would increase greatly, and the possibility of viable tissue preservation in the ischemic penumbra would decrease, if recanalization occurs later.

Tissue Plasminogen Activator and Single-Chain Urokinase Plasminogen Activator

The activities of the agents tPA and scuPA appear unique. Therefore, a consideration of their specific properties, their use in some clinical situations, and their possible use in the setting of acute thrombotic stroke is relevant to the issue of acute stroke treatment (Table 1).

tPA

The agent tPA is a 70000-dalton serine protease, synthesized and secreted by vascular endothelial cells, which possesses relative fibrin specificity capable of lysing fibrin-containing thrombi. It is found in human uterine tissues and is produced constitutively by some tumors including certain human melanomas from which it has been isolated and purified [7, 81, 82]. Purified m-tPA from the cell-free medium of a stable melanoma cell line (RPMI 7272) has properties identical to recombinant tPA (r-tPA) produced by recombinant DNA techniques [81, 83]. The molecule exists in both single- and two-chain forms. The natural molecule is glycosylated at four asparagine sites, contains 527 amino acids, and has two kringle structures [84]. The latter share sequence and structural homology with similar regions on plasminogen, urokinase, and prothrombin [85]. The finger do-

Table 1. Endogenous thrombolytic agents

	tPA	scuPA/urokinase
Molecular weight	70×10^3 daltons	$54-55 \times 10^3$, 31×10^3 daltons
pI	7.5	8.5 – 9.5
Amino acids	527	411
Kringle structures	2	1
Polyeptide chains[a]	1	1[b]
	2 (plasmin)	2 (plasmin)
Activity	1 chain = 2 chain	1 chain < 2 chain
Fibrin binding	1 chain = 2 chain	1 chain = ?, 2 chain = no
Stimulation of activity	Fibrin (1 chain and 2 chain) ↑plasminogen affinity	Fibrin (chain[b] only) neutralizes competitive inhibitor

[a] tPA exists as a single-chain in native form, but may be converted to a two-chain form by limited proteolysis by plasmin. The fibrin-binding affinity and plasminogen activation kinetic rates are roughly equal. In contrast, scuPA exists as a single chain of molecular weight $54-55 \times 10^3$ daltons, which is converted to two-chain urokinase by plasmin. Single-chain (or low molecular weight) urokinase has a molecular weight of 31×10^3 daltons, lacks fibrin affinity and, like two-chain urokinase, mediates systemic plasminogen activation.
[b] scuPA
tPA, tissue plasminogen activator; scuPA, single chain urokinase plasminogen activator

main of tPA has been assumed to be the fibrin recognition and binding site of the molecule.

The native single-chain molecule is converted to the two-chain form by limited digestion by plasmin, which probably occurs in the thrombus [86, 87]. Although the one-chain and two-chain forms have nearly identical fibrinolytic properties, the in vivo fibrinolytic activity is probably due to the two-chain form. The latter form consists of a heavy chain containing the two kringles, while the light chain contains the active site which is responsible for plasminogen cleavage (activation). In vitro studies have demonstrated that the activation of plasminogen to plasmin is accelerated significantly by tPA in the presence of fibrin in the thrombus [83]. Although fibrinogen also stimulates tPA activation of plasminogen, the level of stimulation is considerably less, therefore the designation of tPA as a relatively fibrin-specific agent. The general effect of fibrin-bound tPA is apparently to increase the favorable binding of plasminogen to fibrin and its subsequent activation to plasmin in association with fibrin. tPA thereby increases the local concentration of plasminogen. Interestingly, fibrinogenolysis suggesting activation of plasminogen in the circulation occurs only at high doses at tPA. Whether the fibrinogen breakdown observed in some studies represents an in vitro assay artefact or is dependent upon the type of tPA is a matter of current debate.

The efficacy of recombinant tPA has been tested in various animal models and in patients with various thrombotic disorders. Two examples of animal models relevant to this discussion are presented. A jugular-vein thrombosis model in New Zealand white rabbits, in which a ^{125}I-labelled thrombus suspended from a sterile thread was placed in one jugular vein, has been used for pharmacokinetic studies. Dose-rate dependent thrombus dissolution has been produced by urokinase, m-tPA, and r-tPA, however marked reduction in fibrinogen levels occurred only with the urokinase-treated animals [88]. To examine the physiological consequences of thrombus lysis, a dog model of coronary artery thrombotic occlusion has been employed by several laboratories [89]. Thrombus-selective thrombolysis with r-tPA has been demonstrated in this model in which in situ thrombosis was induced by a copper coil advanced by catheter guidance into the left anterior descending artery. The copper coil is thrombogenic, producing acute vascular occlusion within minutes. Following coronary artery occlusion for 1–2 h tPA at 60000 IU/min for 60 min was infused via the intracoronary route or the intravenous route [89]. In addition to clinically relevant findings (e.g., reperfusion arrythmias), PET scans of the left ventricle were made to demonstrate the extent of perfusion ($H_2{}^{15}O$) and metabolic capacity ([^{11}C]palmitate). Restoration of perfusion was virtually complete and only a minimal residual metabolic defect was apparent following tPA-mediated thrombolysis 1.5 h following coronary artery occlusion. In these and other studies r-tPA has been unequivocably shown to mediate thrombus dissolution in vivo in animal models.

A similar experience in patients has been acquired. The TIMI I trial, a double-blind comparison of intravenous r-tPA and streptokinase within 4 h of the onset of acute MI, demonstrated nearly equal coronary artery perfusion rates after infusion of the two agents [41, 42]. Hemorrhagic complications were not significantly different. Subsequent studies with higher dose rates of r-tPA have been reported to result in a higher frequency of coronary artery patency and perfusion. Whether this approach will result in a decrease in associated mortality remains to be seen. Recently r-tPA has been employed in an angiographic study of acute pulmonary arterial occlusion, or pulmonary embolus [90]. In a well controlled prospective study of 17 patients with acute pulmonary embolus, 16 patients demonstrated pulmonary artery perfusion following tPA infusion, with only one major hemorrhage. Again, any significant effect upon mortality must await a more extensive placebo or therapy controlled study.

At this time, r-tPA has not been used in any controlled study of acute thrombotic stroke.

scuPA and Urokinase

Less experience is available with single-chain urokinase plasminogen activator. This single-chain serine protease has a molecular weight of approximately 55000 daltons and a single internal disulfide linkage. It has been isolated and purified from urine and cell culture medium containing cellular secretions and has been produced in quantity from bacteria by recombinant DNA techniques [7, 91–94]. Limited digestion by plasmin converts scuPA to the two-chain form of urokinase which has an aggregate molecular weight of 55000 and consists of two chains linked by the internal disulfide band. Cleavage of scuPA to form urokinase occurs at lysine (158)-isoleucine (159). Further reduction of the disulfide bridge gives the one-chain form of urokinase (molecular weight 31000), designated as the heavy chain. Both scuPA and two-chain urokinase are enzymatically active and are capable of converting plasminogen to plasmin but have different catalytic properties. Whereas urokinase combines with plasminogen in stoichiometric amounts directly to convert plasminogen to plasmin (which indiscriminantly cleaves fibrinogen and fibrin), scuPA apparently requires fibrin for plasminogen activation. Although the precise mechanism of plasminogen activation by scuPA is unknown, it has been suggested that fibrin displaces or neutralizes a competitive inhibitor attached to scuPA which then allows scuPA to convent plasminogen to plasmin in the presence of fibrin [7, 95]. Fibrinogen does not stimulate the action of scuPA or plasminogen, therefore scuPA is regarded as a relatibvely fibrin-selective agent.

In vitro studies confirm the dose-rate dependence of thrombus dissolution by scuPA, and animal studies in both the rabbit jugular-vein thrombus model and the canine myocardial infarction model have demonstrated the ability of scuPA to lyse fibrin-containing thrombi in vivo [92, 96].

This agent has been employed intravenously in a small number of patients presenting with acute myocardial ischemia, resulting in a return of coronary artery flow in the obstructed vessels (Collen, personal communication). Preliminary experience in this and other discorders has been, to date, quite limited. The process of production and purification of scuPA is significantly less complicated than that of r-tPA, so that for scuPA cost and quantity should be favorable.

tPA and scuPA – Synergism?

Of major interest currently is the observation that r-tPA and scuPA may act together synergistically to produce more efficient thrombolysis than the sum of the activities of each agent taken separately. Although the activities of r-tPA and scuPA appear additive in vitro, in the rabbit model they clearly act synergistically to produce thrombus dissolution [97]. The exact mechanism of synergism is unknown. Although the practical significance may be that much lower quantities of each agent could be necessary to dissolve fibrin thrombi if used together than if use alone, the more interesting problems are whether this combination will produce the fibrinogen degradation observed with very high doses of one preparation of r-tPA in patients and whether the combination of r-tPA and scuPA may be more suitable for thrombotic occlusions in one vascular bed and not another.

It should be remembered that the current clinical experience with urokinase, r-tPA, and scuPA in other disorders is measured against the success of thrombolytic agents to return flow in occluded coronary arteries in patients presenting with acute myocardial infarction.

Application of These Approaches to Acute Stroke

A discussion of the possible utility of the new endogenous thrombolytic agents, tPA and scuPA, in the treatment of acute stroke must take into account the fact that there is no successful standard treatment modality for acute stroke at present. Limited experience with local application of the fibrinolytic agents urokinase and streptokinase within 6–10 h of the onset of acute symptoms of thrombotic occlusion in the carotid and the vertebrobasilar territories has demonstrated that occlusions can be removed in the presence of such agents [1, 74–79]. There is an indication that the clinical outcome in patients who recanalized may have been improved by such therapy. Certainly, patients with acute deficits either did not improve or expired when recanalization was not achieved. The technical and logistical difficulties in many neurological centers of coordinating local intraarterial thrombolysis in acute stroke by interventional neuroradiological techniques suggest that while this approach is the most promising one currently available, certain refinements of this approach are necessary. To test adequately the hypothesis that early lysis of thrombotic occlusions in the appropriate territory can lead to less severe residual neurological deficits and a limitation of the infarction-zone size following an acute thrombotic stroke, a thrombolytic agent which can be readily and safely applied, and appropriate methods for quantitating outcome must be used.

The theoretical and practical advantages of tPA and scuPA are worth mentioning in this regard:

1. Both agents have relative fibrin specificity, thereby producing thrombus selectivity (confining enzymatic action to the fibrin thrombus). Consequently both agents may be applied intravenously, rather then locally.
2. In the case of tPA, except at high systemic doses, fibrinogen is spared so that a hypofibrinogenemic state is note produced.
3. The anticoagulant phase produced by urokinase and streptokinase is not evident with tPA and scuPA. Therefore, it is assumed that the risk of hemorrhage associated with the anticoagulant state may be reduced.
4. Clinical studies in acute stroke may take advantage of experience in patients with acute myocardial infarction regarding reperfusion, kinetics, and specimen handling.
5. Protocols for the study of thrombolysis in acute stroke with the new agents may take advantage of pilot studies conducted with conventional agents administered locally in acute stroke, and of studies of fibrinolysis in acute myocardial infarction.
6. The agents tPA and scuPA may act synergistically.

Certain current limitations of this approach based upon the characteristics of tPA and scuPA, and the natural history of thrombotic stroke must be considered:

1. Like other thrombolytic agents the duration of action of tPA and scuPA is based upon individual factors, e.g., the size, age, and location of the thrombus, which may be largely unknown.
2. The risk of hemorrhage from these agents derivses from lysis of thrombi protecting sites of vascular injury, rather than the anticoagulant state. Therefore, the risk of intracerebral hemorrhage following acute stroke and tPA infusion, for instance, is unknown in a given individual.
3. The incidence of hemorrhagic infarction and parenchymatous hemorrhage following acute thrombotic stroke in the absence of therapy is largely unknown. Various estimates range from 0%–43% in clinical studies [98–108], and 60%–70% in postmortem studies [109, 110].
4. The dose-rate for tPA in acute stroke necessary to lyse thrombotic occlusions is unknown.

5. The peculiar flow characteristics of the circle of Willis may be important in the success of fibrinolysis in the carotid territory. With proximal MCA occlusion, lysis of the thrombus does not occur when urokinase is infused at the carotid bifurcation, presumably because of flow of the agent into the anterior and posterior cerebral territories. It is unknown whether more effective lysis of proximal MCA occlusions can be achieved by systemic or direct superselective application of substances such as tPA, however, this must be carefully studied.
6. Previous studies have suggested that with the practical limitations of acquiring patients early, the effect of thrombolytic therapy is most probably directed at reducing the ischemic region in the "ischemic penumbra."

These limitations suggest caution in future studies with tPA and/or scuPA in acute stroke. Rather than being a liability, the unknowns suggested should be used as the basis for the careful design of clinical protocols to test the hypothesis with tPA. Such protocols in preparation for a multicenter study of the safety and efficacy of fibrin-selective thrombolytic agents in acute thrombotic stroke have been designed. In addition, valuable information regarding various aspects of acute thrombotic stroke can be obtained.

Rash and unreasoned use of these agents in acute thrombotic stroke at this stage of development may have the effect of negating a potentially useful approach.

References

1. del Zoppo GJ, Zeumer H, Harker LA (1986) Thrombolytic therapy in acute stroke: Possibilities and hazards. Stroke 17:595–607
2. Kakkar VV, Scully MF (1978) Thrombolytic therapy. Br Med Bull 34:191–199
3. Sharma GVRK, Cella G, Parish AF, Sasahara AA (1982) Drug therapy: thrombolytic therapy. N Engl J Med 306:1268–1276
4. Verstraete M (1978) Biochemical and clinical aspects of thrombolysis. Semin Hematol 15:35–54
5. Bachmann F, Kruithof IEKO (1984) Tissue plasminogen activator: chemical and physiological aspects. Semin Thromb Hemost 10:6–17
6. Collen D, Lijnen HR (1984) New approaches to thrombolytic therapy. Arteriosclerosis 4:579–585
7. Verstraete M, Collen D (1986) Thrombolytic therapy in the eighties. Blood 67:1529–1541
8. Thompson AR, Harker LA (1983) Manual of hemostasis and thrombosis. Davis, Philadelphia, pp 41–45
9. Kaplan AP (1978) Initiation of the intrinsic coagulation and fibrinolytic pathways of man: the role of surfaces, Hageman factor, prekallikrein, high molecular weight kininogen, and factor XI. Prog Hemost Thromb 4:127
10. Hermans J, McDonagh J (1982) Fibrin: structure and interactions. Semin Thromb Hemost 8:11–24
11. Castellino FJ (1984) Biochemistry of human plasminogen. Semin Thromb Hemost 10:18–23
12. Walsh P, Greenspan RH, Simon AL (1978) Urokinase-pulmonary embolism trial. Circulation 67 (suppl):1–108
13. Urokinase Streptokinase Embolism Trial (1974) JAMA 16:1606–1613
14. Dotter CT, Seaman AJ (1974) Clot lysis with low-dose streptokinase. Radiology 111:31–37
15. Katzen BT, van Breda A (1981) Low dose streptokinase in the treatment of arterial occlusions. Am J Radiol 136:1171–1181
16. Hess H, Ingrisch H, Mietaschk A, Rath H (1982) Local low-dose thrombolytic therapy of peripheral arterial occlusions. N Engl J Med 307:1627–1630

17. Verstraete M (1972) Thrombolytic treatment of recent arterial occlusion. J Clin Pathol 25:641–642
18. Poliwoda H, Alexander K, Buhl V, Holsten D, Wagner HH (1969) Treatment of chronic arterial occlusions with streptokinase. N Engl J Med 280:689–692
19. Hume M, Gurewich V, Thomas DP, Dealy Jr JB (1970) Streptokinase for chronic arterial occlusive disease. Arch Surg 101:653–657
20. Poliwoda H (1972) Treatment of chronic arterial occlusions with streptokinase. J Clin Pathol 27:642–643
21. Reichle FA, Rao NS, Chang KHY, Marder V, Algazy K (1977) Thrombolysis of acute or subacute non-embolic arterial thrombosis. J Surg Res 22:202–208
22. Martin M, Roth F-J, Fiebach BJO, Auel H (1978) Fibrinolytische Therapie mit Aktivator. Dtsch Med Wochenschr 103:1953–1957
23. Martin M, Auel H (1979) Thrombolytic therapy in arterial thromboembolism. Prog Cardiovasc Dis XXI(5):351–374
24. Rentrop P, Blanke H, Weigand V, Karsch KR (1979) Wiederöffnung verschlossener Kranzgefäße im akuten Infarkt mit Hilfe von Kathetern (Transluminale Rekanalisation). Dtsch Med Wochenschr 104:1401
25. Rentrop P, Blanke H, Karsch KR, Kaeser H, Kostering H, Leitz K (1981) Selective intracoronary thrombolysis in acute myocardial infarction and unstable angina pectoris. Circulation 63:307–317
26. Mathey DG, Kuck K-H, Tilsner V, Krebber H-J, Bleifeld W (1981) Nonsurgical coronary artery recanalization in acute transmural myocardial infarction. Circulation 63:489–497
27. Ganz W, Buchbinder N, Marcus H, Mondkar A, Maddahi J, Chruzi Y, O'Connor L, Shell W, Fishbein MC, Kass R, Miyamoto A, Swan JHC (1981) Intracoronary thrombolysis in evolving myocardial infarction. Am Heart J 101:4–13
28. Cowley MJA, Hastillo A, Vetrovec GW, Hess ML (1981) Effects of intracoronary streptokinase in acute myocardial infarction. Am Heart J 10:1149–1158
29. Neuhaus KL, Tebbe U, Sauer G, Rahlf G, Kostering H, Kreuzer K (1981) High-dose i.v. streptokinase infusion in acute myocardial infarction. Eur Heart J 2:144
30. Rutsch W, Schartl M, Mathey D, Kuck K, Merx W, Dorr R, Rentrop P, Blanke H (1981) Percutaneous transluminal coronary recanalization: Procedure, results, and acute complications. Am Heart J 102:1178–1181
31. Ganz W, Geft I, Maddahi J, Berman D, Charuzi Y, Shah PK, Swan HJC (1983) Non-surgical reperfusion in evolving myocardial infarction. J Am Coll Cardiol 1:1247–1253
32. Timmis GC, Gangadharan V, Hauser AM, Ramos RG, Westveer DC, Gordon S (1982) Intracoronary streptokinase in clinical practice. Am Heart J 104:925–938
33. Smalling RW, Fuentes F, Freund GC, Reduto LA, Wanta-Matthews M, Gaeta JM, Walker W, Sterling R, Gould KL (1982) Beneficial effects of intracoronary thrombolysis up to eighteen hours after onset of pain in evolving myocardial infarction. Am Heart J 104:912–920
34. Khaja F, Walton Jr JA, Brymer JF, Lo E, Osterberger L, O'Neil WW, Colfer HT, Weiss R, Lee T, Kurian T, Goldberg AD, Pitt B, Goldstein S (1983) Intracoronary fibrinolytic therapy in acute myocardial infarction. N Engl J Med 308:1305–1311
35. Anderson JL, Marshall HW, Bray BE, Lutz JR, Frederick PR, Yanowitz FG, Datz FL, Klausner SC, Hagan AD (1983) A randomized trial of intracoronary streptokinase in the treatment of acute myocardial infarction. N Engl J Med 308:1312–1318
36. Kennedy JW, Ritchie JL, Davis KB, Fritz JK (1983) Western Washington randomized trial of intracoronary streptokinase in acute myocardial infarction. N Engl J Med 309:1477–1482
37. Leiboff RH, Katz RJ, Wasserman AG, Bren GB, Schwartz H, Varghese J, Ross AM (1984) A randomized, angiographically controlled trial of intracoronary streptokinase in acute myocardial infarction. Am J Cardiol 53:404–407
38. Schroeder R, Biamino G, Leitner E-R, Linderer T, Bruggemann T, Heitz J, Vohringer H-F, Wegscheider K (1983) Intravenous short-term infusion of streptokinase in acute myocardial infarction. Circulation 67:536–548
39. Spann JF, Sherry S, Carabello BA, Denenberg BS, Mann RH, McCann WD, Gault JH, Gentzler RD, Belber AD, Maurer AH, Copper EM (1984) Coronary thrombolysis by intravenous streptokinase in acute myocardial infarction: acute and follow-up studies. Am J Cardiol 53:655–661
40. European Cooperative Study Group (1979) Streptokinase in acute myocardial infarction. N Engl J Med 301:797–802

41. TIMI Study Group (1985) Special report: The thrombolysis in myocardial infarction (TIMI) trial. N Engl J Med 312:932–936
42. Aber CP, Bass NM, Berry CL, Carson PHM, Dobbs RJ, Fox KM, Hamblin JJ, Haydu SP, Howitt G, MacIver JE, Portal RW, Raftery EB, Rousell RH, Stock JPP (1976) Streptokinase in acute myocardial infarction: a controlled multicentre study in the United Kingdom. Br Med J 2:1100–1104
43. Robertson BR, Nilsson IM, Nylander G, Olow B (1967) Effect of streptokinase and heparin on patients with deep venous thrombosis. Acta Chir Scand 133:205–215
44. Robertson BR, Nilsson IM, Nylander G (1968) Value of streptokinase and heparin in treatment of acute deep venous thrombosis. Acta Chir Scand 134:203–208
45. Kakkar VV, Flanc C, O'Shea MJ, Flute PT, Howe CT, Clarke MB (1969) Treatment of deep-vein thrombosis with streptokinase. Br J Surg 56:178–183
46. Mavor GE, Bennett B, Galloway JMD, Karmody AM (1969) Streptokinase in iliofemoral venous thrombosis. Br J Surg 56:564–570
47. Mavor GE, Dhall DP, Dawson AA, Duthie JS, Walker MG, Mahaffy RG, Allardyce M (1973) Streptokinase therapy in deep-vein thrombosis. Br J Surg 60:468–474
48. Tsapogas MJ, Peabody RA, Wu KT, Karmody AM, Devaraj KT, Eckert C (1973) Controlled study of thrombolytic therapy in deep vein thrombosis. Surgery 74:973–984
49. Astedt B, Robertson B, Haeger K (1974) Experience with standardized streptokinase therapy of depp venous thrombosis. Surg Gynecol Obstet 139:387–388
50. Chavatzas D, Martin P (1975) A study of streptokinase in deep vein thrombosis of the lower extremities. Vasa 4:68–72
51. Duckert F, Muller G, Nyman D, Benz A, Prisender S, Madar G, Da Silva MA, Widmer LK, Schmitt HE (1975) Treatment of deep vein thrombosis with streptokinase. Br Med J 1:479–481
52. Kakkar VV, Lewis M, Sagar S (1975) Treatment of deep-vein thrombosis with intermittent streptokinase and plasminogen infusion. Lancet i:674–676
53. Marder VJ, Loulen RL, Atichartakarn V, Budzynski AZ, Parulekar S, Kim JR, Edward N, Zahavi J, Algazy KM (1977) Quantitative venographic assessment of deep vein thrombosis in the evaluation of streptokinase and heparin therapy. J Lab Clin Med 89:1018–1029
54. Seaman AJ, Common HH, Rosch J, Dotter CT, Porter JM, Lindell TD, Lawler WL, Schlueter WJ (1976) Deep vein thrombosis treated with streptokinase or heparin: a randomized study. Angiology 27:549–556
55. Bieger R, Boekhout-Mussert RJ, Hohmann F, Loeliger EA (1976) Is streptokinase useful in the treatment of deep vein thrombosis? Acta Med Scand 199:81–88
56. Arnesen H, Heilo A, Jakobsen E, Ly B, Skaga E (1978) A prospective study of streptokinase and heparin in the treatment of deep vein thrombosis. Acta Med Scand 203:457–463
57. Jarvinen P, Aromaa U, Roiha M, Asp K (1978) Streptokinase and concomitant oral anticoagulants in the treatment of deep venous thrombosis. Klin Wochenschr 56:801–804
58. Marbet GA, Eichlisberger R, Duckert F, de Silva MA, Biland L, Widmer LK, Ritz R, Schmitt HE (1982) Sequential treatment of deep leg vein thrombosis with porcine plasmin and low dose streptokinase. Thromb Haemost 48:190–195
59. Schulman S, Lockner D, Granqvist S, Bratt G, Paul C, Nyman D (1984) A comparative randomized trial of low-dose versus high-dose streptokinase in deep vein thrombosis of the thigh. Thromb Haemost 51:261–265
60. Trubestein G (1984) Indikation und Durchführung der fibrinolytischen Therapie mit Streptokinase und Urokinase bei tiefer Venenthrombose. Vasa (Suppl) 12:104–113
61. Serradimigni A, Bory M, Dijiane P, Mathieu P, Leonetti J, Juhan-Vague I, Sampol J (1978) Treatment of venous thrombosis and pulmonary embolism by streptokinase. Angiology 29:825–831
62. Sherry S (1985) Tissue plasminogen activator (t-PA): will it fulfill its promise? N Engl J Med 313:1014–1017
63. Marder VJ (1986) Fibrinolytic agents: are they feasible for stroke therapy? In: Plum F, Pulsinelli WA (eds) Cerebrovascular diseases, fourteenth research conference. Raven, New York, pp 241–247
64. Cercek B, Lew AS, Hod H, Yano J, Reddy NKN, Ganz W (1986) Enhancement of thrombolysis with tissue-type plasminogen activator by pretreatment with heparin. Circulation 74:583–587
65. Solis OJ, Roberson GR, Taveras JM, Mohr J, Pessin MS (1977) Cerebral angiography in acute cerebral infarction. Revist Interam Radiol 2:19–25

66. Clarke RL, Cliffton EE (1960) The treatment of cerebrovascular thrombosis and embolism with fibrinolytic agents. Am J Cardiol 30:546–551
67. Meyer JS, Herndon RM, Gotoh F, Tazaki Y, Nelson JN, Johnson JF (1961) Therapeutic thrombolysis. In: Millikan CH, Siekert RG, Whisnant JP (eds) Cerebral vascular disease, third princeton conference. Grune and Stratton, New York, pp 160–177
68. Herndon RM, Nelson JN, Johnson JF, Meyer JS (1961) Thrombolytic treatment in cerebrovascular thrombosis. In: MacMillan RL, Mustard JF (eds) Anticoagulants and fibrinolysins, Lea and Febiger, Philadelphia, pp 154–164
69. Meyer JS, Gilroy J, Barnhart ME, Johnson JF (1965) Therapeutic thrombolysis in cerebral thromboembolism: randomized evaluation of intravenous streptokinase. In: Millikan CH, Siekert RG, Whisnant JP (eds). Cerebral vascular diseases, fourth princeton conference. Grune and Stratton, New York, pp 200–213
70. Fletcher AP, Alkjaersig N, Lewis M, Tulevski V, Davies A, Brooks JE, Mardin WB, Landau WM, Raichle ME (1976) A pilot study of urokinase therapy in cerebral infarction. Stroke 7:135–142
71. Hanaway J, Torack R, Fletcher AP, Landau WM (1976) Intracranial bleeding associated with urokinase therapy for acute ischemic hemispheral stroke. Stroke 7:143–146
72. Kaufman HH, Lind TA, Clark DS (1977) Non-penetrating trauma to the carotid artery with secondary thrombosis and embolism: treatment by thrombolysin. Acta Neurochir 37:219–244
73. Atkin N, Nitzberg S, Dorsey J (1964) Lysis of intracerebral thromboembolism with fibrinolysin. Angiology 15:436–439
74. Matuso O, Kosugi T, Mihara H, Ohki Y, Matsuo T (1979) Retrospective study on the efficacy of using urokinase therapy. Acta Haematol 42:684–688
75. Abe T, Kazawa M, Naito I (1981) Clinical effect of urokinase (60000 units/day) on cerebral infarction-comparative study by means of multiple center double blind test. Blood Vessels 12:342–358
76. Abe T, Kazawa M, Naito I (1981) Clinical evaluation for efficacy of tissue culture urokinase (TCUK) on cerebral thrombosis by means of multicenter double-blind study. Blood Vessels 12:321–341
77. Nenci GG, Gresele P, Taramelli M, Agnelli G, Signorini E (1983) Thrombolytic therapy for thromboembolism of vertebrobasilar artery. Angiology 34:561–571
78. Miyakawa T (1984) The cerebral vessels and thrombosis. Rinsho Ketsueki 25:1018–1026
79. Zeumer H (1985) Survey of progress: vascular recanalizing techniques in interventional neuroradiology. J Neurol 231:287–294
80. Bruckmann H, Ferbert A, del Zoppo GJ, Hacke W, Zeumer H (1987) The acute vertebrobasilar thrombosis: angiological-clinical comparison and therapeutic implications. Acta Radiol 369:38–42
81. Rijken DC, Collen D (1981) Purification and characterization of the plasminogen activator secreted by human melanoma cells in culture. J Biol Chem 256:7035
82. Ranby M (1982) Tissue plasminogen activator. Isolation, enzymatic properties and assay procedure. Thesis, Umea University, Umea, Medical Dissertations New Series, no. 90:7035
83. Zamarron C, Lijnen HR, Collen D (1984) Kinetics of the activation of plasminogen by natural and recombinant tissue-type plasminogen activator. J Biol Chem 259:2080–2083
84. Pennica D, Holmes WE, Kohr WJ, Harkins RN, Vehar GA, Ward CA, Bennett WF, Yelverton E, Seeburg PH, Heyneker HL, Goeddel DV, Collen D (1983) Cloning and expression of human tissue-type plasminogen activator cDNA in E. coli. Nature 301:214
85. Strassburger W, Wollmer A, Pitts JE, Glover ID, Tickle IJ, Blundell TL, Steffens GJ, Gunzler WA, Otting F, Flohe L (1983) Adaptation of plasminogen activator sequences to known protease structures. FEBS Lett 157:219
86. Rijken DC, Hoylaerts M, Collen D (1982) Fibrinolytic properties of one-chain and two-chain human extrinsic (tissue-type) plasminogen activator. J Biol Chem 257:2920
87. Ranby M, Bergsdorf N, Nilsson T (1982) Enzymatic properties of the one- and two-chain form of tissue plasminogen activator. Thromb Res 27:175
88. Collen D, Stassen JM, Marafino Jr BJ, Buildeo S, de Cock F, Ogez J, Tajiri D, Pennica D, Bennett WF, Saliva J, Hoyng CF (1984) Biological properties of human tissue-type plasminogen activator obtained by expression of recombinant DNA in mammalian cells. J Physiol Exp Ther 231:146–152
89. Bergmann SR, Fox KAA, Ter-Pogossian MM, Sobel BE, Collen D (1983) Clot-selective coronary thrombolysis with tissue-type plasminogen activator. Science 220:1181–1183

90. Goldhaber SZ, Vaughan DE, Markis JE, Selwyn AP, Meyerovitz M, Loscalzo J, Dawley DL, Sharma GVRK, Sasahara A, Grossbard EB, Braunwald E (1986) Efficacy and safety of tissue plasminogen activator in treatment of acute pulmonary embolism. In: VIIIthe international congress on fibrinolysis, Wien
91. Gunzler WA, Steffens GJ, Otting F, Kim SMA, Frankus E, Flohe L (1982) The primary structure of high molecular mass urokinase from human urine. Hoppe-Seyler's Z Physiol Chem 363:1155–1165
92. Husain S, Gurewich V, Lipinski B (1983) Purification and partial characterization of a single-chain high-molecular-weight form of urokinase from human urine. Arch Biochem Biophys 220:31
93. Collen D, Zamarron C, Lijnen HR, Hoylaerts M (1986) Activation of plasminogen by pro-urokinase. II. Kinetics. J Biol Chem 261:1253
94. Zamarron C, Lijnen HR, Van Hoef B, Collen D (1984) Biological and thrombolytic properties of proenzyme and active forms of human urokinase. I. Fibrinolytic and fibrinogenolytic properties in human plasma in vitro of urokinase obtained from human urine or by recombinant DNA technology. Thromb Haemost 52:19
95. Lijnen HR, Zamarron C, Collen D (1985) Pro-urokinase: kinetics and mechanism of action. Thromb Haemost 54(suppl 1):118
96. Collen D, Stump D, Van de Werf F, Jang IK, Nobuhara M, Lijnen HR (1985) Coronary thrombolysis in dogs with intravenously administered human pro-urokinase. Circulation 72:384
97. Collen D (1986) Human tissue-type plasminogen activator (t-PA) and single chain urokinase-type plasminogen activator (scu-PA) act synergically on clot lysis in vivo but not in vitro. In: VIIIth international congress on fibrinolysis, Wien
98. Hornig CR, Dorndorf W, Agnoli AL (1986) Hemorrhagic cerebral infarction: a prospective study. Stroke 17:179–185
99. Mohr JP, Caplan LR, Melski JW, Golstein RJ, Duncan GW, Kistler JP, Pessin MS, Bleich HL (1978) The Harvard Cooperative Stroke registry: a prospective registry. Neurology 28:754–762
100. Aring CD, Merritt HH (1935) Differential diagnosis between cerebral hemorrhage and cerebral thrombosis. Arch Intern Med 56:435–456
101. Whisnant JP, Fitzgibbons JP, Kurland LT (1971) Natural history of stroke in Rochester, Minnesota, 1945 through 1954. Stroke 2:11–22
102. Matsumoto N, Whisnant JP, Kurland LT (1973) Natural history of stroke in Rochester, Minnesota, 1955 through 1969: an extension of previous study, 1945 through 1954. Stroke 4:20–29
103. Kannel WB, Dawber TR, Cohen MS (1973) Vascular disease of the brain – epidemiologic aspects: the Framingham study. Am J Public Health 63:53–58
104. Wells CE (1959) Cerebral embolism: The natural history, prognostic signs, and effects of anticoagulation. AMA Arch Neurol Psychiatr 81:667–677
105. Howell DA, Tatlow TWF, Feldman S (1964) Observations on anticoagulant therapy in thromboembolic disease of the brain. Can Med Assoc J 90:611–614
106. Carter AB (1965) Prognosis of cerebral embolism. Lancet ii:514–519
107. De Wit H, Wise RA (1977) Blockade of cocaine reinforcement in rats with the dopamine receptor blocker pimozide, but not with the noradrenergic blockers phentolamine and phenoxybenzamine. Can J Psychol 31:195–203
108. Baker RN, Broward JA, Fang HC, Fisher CM, Groch SN, Heyman A, Karp HR, McDevitt E, Scheinberg P, Schwartz W, Toole JF (1962) Anaticoagulant therapy in cerebral infarction. Neurology 12:823–835
109. Fisher CM, Adams RD (1951) Observations on brain embolism with special reference to the mechanism of hemorrhagic infarction. J Neuropathol Exp Neurol 10:92–94
110. Jorgensen L, Torvik A (1969) Ischaemic cerebrovascular diseases in an autopsy series. Part 2. Prevalence, location, pathogenesis, and clinical course of cerebral infarcts. J Neurol Sci 9:285–320

Calcium Antagonists and Other Cerebroprotective Drugs

J. KRIEGLSTEIN[1], G. W. BIELENBERG[1], and H.-J. STIERSTORFER[1]

There are many drugs offered on the market to protect brain against ischemic damage and to improve brain function after ischemic attacks. Calcium antagonists and calcium-entry blockers are a group of drugs which seems to be most prominent in this respect. Therefore, the discussion of the effects to calcium-entry blockers assumes a large part of this presentation, although certain other drugs will also be discussed.

Calcium-entry blockers are widely investigated as cerebroprotective drugs because they evince distinct pharmacological activity and because their mechanism of action is relatively clear. Their essential effect is to inhibit the influx of Ca^{2+} through the voltage-operated calcium channels. Under normal conditions this effect leads, for instance, to a relaxation of smooth muscle cells or to an inhibition of transmitter release in neurons. Under pathophysiological conditions of energy failure the cytosol of cells may be flooded by Ca^{2+}, because the high Ca^{2+} concentration gradient (about 1 mmol Ca^{2+}/l in the extracellular space and about 0.1 µmol Ca^{2+}/l in the cytosol) can no longer be maintained. The cytosolic concentration of Ca^{2+} increases tremendously and triggers a cascade of reactions (Fig. 1) which may lead finally to cell necrosis. Applying calcium-entry blockers to such a situation of energy failure in brain tissue could mean that the Ca^{2+} influx is reduced, the cascade of consequent reactions is inhibited and the neuronal necrosis may be prevented.

The question here regards which sort of cells in the brain do calcium entry blockers act upon. Do these act only upon smooth-muscle cells of brain vessels, or do they also act upon neurons? It is difficult to differentiate between these effects in the rat brain in vivo. We have therefore used the isolated perfused rat brain, which offers clear-cut experimental conditions [4, 5].

A fluorocarbon emulsion was used as perfusion medium and drugs were added to this medium before perfusion was started. The EEG of the isolated brain, which was not different from that obtained from rat brain in vivo, was recorded during the entire experimental period. After a preperfusion period of 30 min, perfusion was stopped for 30 min (= ischemia) and continued thereafter for various time periods (= reperfusion). At the end of the experiment the isolated brains were immersed in liquid nitrogen, the cortical tissue was dissected at −20 °C and extracted with methanolic HCl and perchloric acid (0.3 mol/l). Substrates of energy metabolism were measured enzymatically in this extract [3].

[1] Institute of Pharmacology and Toxicology, FB 16, Philipps-University, Ketzerbach 63, D-3550 Marburg, FRG

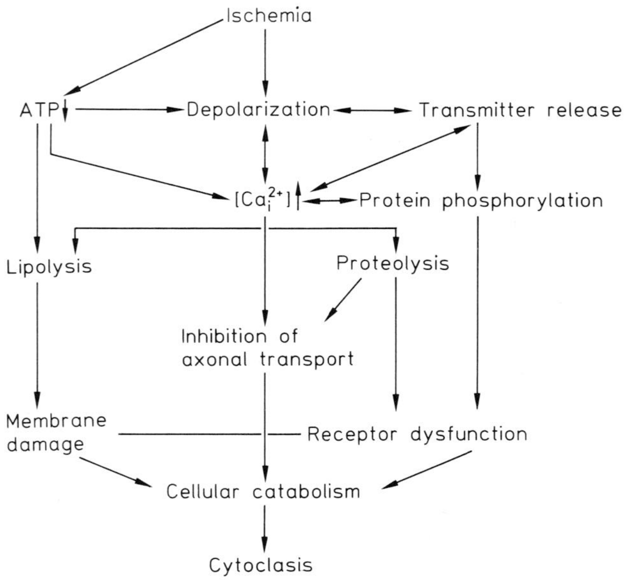

Fig. 1. Cascade of reactions caused by brain ischemia. (According to Siesjö and Wieloch 1985)

Table 1. Effect of nimodipine on the energy state in the cortical tissue of the isolated perfused rat brain

Substrate	Control (n = 6)	Nimodipine (n = 7)
Phosphocreatine	0.39 ± 0.37	2.61 ± 1.26***
ATP	0.51 ± 0.09	1.68 ± 0.23***
ADP	0.69 ± 0.05	0.52 ± 0.09***
AMP	1.36 ± 0.31	0.39 ± 0.22***
Total adenylate	2.56 ± 0.29	2.59 ± 0.13
Energy charge	0.34 ± 0.06	0.75 ± 0.09***
Glucose	0.34 ± 0.11	0.34 ± 0.21
Glucose 6-phosphate	0.009 ± 0.006	0.055 ± 0.036***
Fructose 1,6-diphosphate	0.028 ± 0.010	0.055 ± 0.023**
Pyruvate	0.015 ± 0.010	0.081 ± 0.032***
Lactate	8.4 ± 1.0	7.3 ± 0.5*
Lactate/pyruvate	642.4 ± 318.2	104.8 ± 46.1***

Experimental conditions: 30 min preperfusion + 30 min ischemia + 5 min reperfusion. Nimodipine was added to the perfusion medium at a concentration of 0.5 μmol/l. Values are given as mean ± SD in μmol/g cortical tissue (wet weight).
Energy charge = ATP + 1/2 ADP/ATP + ADP + AMP.
For statistical comparisons Student's t test was used: *$p<0.05$, **$p<0.01$, ***$p<0.001$

Table 1 shows the influence of nimodipine on energy metabolism of the isolated rat brain after 5 min of reperfusion. The levels of the high-energy phosphates ATP and phosphocreatine (among others) were higher in drug-treated than in control cortical tissue, while the lactate level and the lactate/pyruvate ratio were lower.

In order to interpret these results it was necessary to obtain information on the effect of nimodipine on cerebral blood flow under the same experimental con-

Table 2. Effect of nimodipine on postischemic hypoperfusion of the isolated rat brain

	Perfusion rate (ml/min)	
	Control ($n = 6$)	Nimodipine ($n = 7$)
Preperfusion		
5 min	4.3 ± 0.4	4.8 ± 0.9
15 min	5.2 ± 0.9	5.1 ± 0.6
30 min	5.0 ± 1.2	4.8 ± 0.5
Reperfusion		
1 min	1.6 ± 0.3	2.9 ± 0.7***

***$p < 0.001$

ditions. As shown in Table 2, nimodipine does not influence blood flow during the preperfusion period but improves the postischemic hypoperfusion. Therefore, we cannot rule out that the increased ATP and phosphocreatine levels may be caused by the increased perfusion rate. However, the reduction of the cortical lactate concentration by nimodipine cannot be explained simply by an increased perfusion rate because lactate is removed in brain tissue to a great extent by metabolism. To shed additional light on this postischemic decrease in the lactate level, which was accelerated by nimodipine, the isolated rat brain was perfused with a calcium-entry blocker at a constant flow rate [1]. The fall in the lactate level during the postischemic period was still accelerated by the drug under these conditions, whereas the drugs effect on the ATP level was abolished.

Therefore, it may be concluded that the improved postischemic hypoperfusion could be responsible for the faster increase in the ATP level, but the postischemia fall of the lactate level seems to be independent of the blood flow and is direct effect of the calcium-entry blocker upon brain parenchyma. Both the effects of calcium-entry blockers on postischemic hypoperfusion and on energy metabolism could protect brain against ischemic damage.

Besides the calcium-entry blockers two further examples or cerebroprotective drugs must be presented. First, naftidrofuryl was studied in the isolated rat brain. Similarly the aforementioned experiments, the isolated rat brain was preperfused for 40 min and after two ischemic periods of 2 min (40th – 42nd min and 50th – 52nd min), this was reperfused for various time periods. When naftidrofuryl was added to the perfusion medium, the EEG of the isolated brain reappeared within 30 s after ischemia, whereas in control brains a spontaneous EEG was again observable only after several minutes. Energy metabolism of the isolated rat brain was also clearly influenced by naftidrofuryl. In particular, the cortical lactate concentration was again significantly reduced by the drug during the postischemio periods (Fig. 2). These experiments clearly demonstrate that naftidrofuryl improves brain function and energy metabolism, at least within the period immediately after ischemia [7].

The last part of this paper represents a somewhat speculative approach. As is known from clinical therapy, drug effects on cerebrovascular diseases may be seen after long-term treatment. It may be argued that the reason for delay in im-

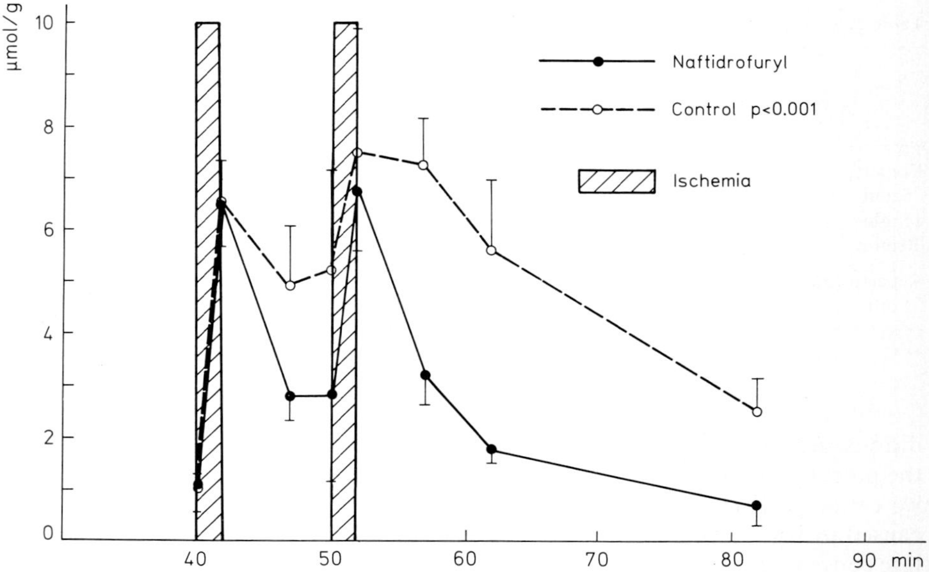

Fig. 2. Influence of naftidrofuryl (10 µmol/l) on the cortical lactate level in the isolated perfused rat brain

provement is the induction of key enzymes of energy metabolism. We attempted to test this hypothesis using rat primary glial cultures. These cells can be derived with high purity and survive for 4–6 weeks in culture. The glial cells were incubated with various cerebroprotective drugs to ascertain whether enzyme induction could occur. Especially the incubation of rat primary glial cells with meclofenoxate for 4 weeks changed the enzymatic pattern remarkably. Most of the enzyme activities measured were significantly changed by the drug: the activity of hexokinase, phosphofructokinase, cytochrome *c* reductase, glucose 6-phosphate dehydrogenase, and malate dehydrogenase were significantly increased, whereas pyruvate kinase activity was reduced and lactate dehydrogenase activity remained unchanged (Table 3; [2]). When, after an incubation period of 3 or 4 weeks, meclofenoxate was withdrawn from the cultured glial cells for 2 or 7 days, some of the drug effects, especially the increased activity of cytochrome *c* reductase, were still measurable (Table 3). It was interesting to discover that meclofenoxate was able also to induce cytochrome *c* reductase in rat brain in vivo when the animals were pretreated with this drug for 4 weeks [2].

In summary, various effects of cerebroprotective drugs on brain circulation, metabolism, and function are demonstrable under experimental conditions. These include the following:

- increase in cerebral blood flow, especially an improvement of postischemic hypoperfusion
- acceleration of ATP resynthesis after ischemia
- accelerated decrease in lactate levels after ischemia
- induction of key enzymes of energy metabolism

Table 3. Influence of meclofenoxate on various enzyme activities in primary rat glial cultures and rat brain in vivo

Enyzme	Treatment	Enzyme Activities			
		Primary rat glial cultures			Rats in vivo
		Incubation 4 weeks	Incubation 4 weeks, deprivation 2 days	Incubation 3 weeks, deprivation 1 week	
Hexokinase	C	36.5 ± 2.4	52.2 ± 3.0	38.3 ± 3.3	5525 ± 556
	T	41.1 ± 2.0*	47.1 ± 2.8*	39.3 ± 2.9	6050 ± 252
Phosphofructokinase	C	57.9 ± 3.2	51.1 ± 6.2	50.3 ± 3.6	11525 ± 2066
	T	71.3 ± 5.6**	59.9 ± 9.9	53.8 ± 2.8	10275 ± 1328
Pyruvate kinase	C	359.7 ± 16.5	425.5 ± 16.9	367.3 ± 30.7	58.5 ± 6.38
	T	317.6 ± 24.3*	413.1 ± 18.8	335.9 ± 14.6	62.4 ± 3.47
Lactate dehydrogenase	C	1.12 ± 0.07	1.21 ± 0.02	1.04 ± 0.02	81.1 ± 9.1
	T	1.15 ± 0.04	1.22 ± 0.05	1.08 ± 0.03	92.3 ± 7.0
Glucose 6-phosphate dehydrogenase	C	125.8 ± 3.0	167.8 ± 7.2	104.4 ± 2.8	23200 ± 2070
	T	162.2 ± 8.0***	232.8 ± 11.1***	130.1 ± 8.4***	25475 ± 1597
Malate dehydrogenase	C	1.34 ± 0.04	1.58 ± 0.04	1.68 ± 0.03	392.1 ± 23.7
	T	1.55 ± 0.05***	1.74 ± 0.04***	1.67 ± 0.03	428.7 ± 46.0
Glutamate dehydrogenase	C	104.2 ± 7.7	146.9 ± 9.7	157.1 ± 5.5	22725 ± 2466
	T	155.2 ± 10.8***	192.8 ± 6.7***	153.9 ± 7.7	25250 ± 1415
Cytochrome *c* reductase	C	72.7 ± 2.0	75.8 ± 5.7	58.7 ± 3.9	3750 ± 532
	T	109.9 ± 4.1***	94.6 ± 8.9**	68.5 ± 5.8*	4875 ± 435*

After an incubation period of 3 or 4 weeks, meclofenoxate (1 mmol/l) was withdrawn from glial cultures for 2 or 7 days. After treatment of male Sprague – Dawley rats with meclosfenoxate (200 ml/kg, i.p., daily for 4 weeks) enzyme activities were measured in cerebral cortical tissues. Values are given as means ± SD of 5 – 6 experiments in mU/mg protein for glial cultures and in U/g wet tissue for cerebral cortex.
For statistical comparisons Student's *t* test was used: *$p<0.05$, **$p<0.01$, ***$p<0.001$.
C, Control; T, Treatment with meclofenoxate

- increased tolerance of hypoxia and ischemia
- accelerated reappearance of the spontaneous EEG after a period of complete ischemia

These drug effects seem to be of interest and of significance. The findings support hypotheses put forward for cerebroprotective mechanisms of action. Nevertheless, the relevance of these effects for drug therapy of cerebrovascular diseases remains to be shown.

References

1. Bielenberg GW, Beck T, Haubruck H, Krieglstein J (1986) Effects of calcium entry blocker emopamil on postischemic energy metabolism of the isolated perfused rat brain and on local cerebral blood flow in the conscious rat. In: Krieglstein J (ed) Pharmacology of cerebral ischemia. Elsevier, Amsterdam
2. Bielenberg GW, Hayn C, Krieglstein J (1986) Effects of cerebro-protective agents on enzyme activities of rat primary glial cultures and rat cerebral cortex. Biochem Pharmacol 35:2693–2702
3. Folbergrova J, Pontén U, Siesjö BK (1974) Patterns of changes in brain carbohydrate metabolites, amino acids and organic phosphates at increased carbon dioxide tensions. J Neurochem 22:1115–1125
4. Hanke J, Krieglstein J (1982) Über die Mechanismen der protektiven Wirkung von Methohexital auf den zerebralen Energiestoffwechsel. Arzneimittel-Forsch 32:620–625
5. Krieglstein G, Krieglstein J, Stock R (1972) Suitability of the isolated perfused rat brain for studying effects on cerebral metabolism. Naunyn-Schmiedeberg's Arch Pharmacol 275:124–134
6. Siesjö BK, Wieloch T (1985) Cerebral metabolism in ischemia: Neurochemical basis for therapy. Br J Anaesth 57:47–62
7. Stierstorfer HJ, Krieglstein J (1986) Effects of naftidrofuryl on postischemic energy metabolism and EEG of the isolated perfused rat brain. In: Krieglstein J (ed) Pharmacology of cerebral ischemia. Elsevier, Amsterdam

Effect of Nimodipine on the Cerebral Circulation and Acute Ischemic Stroke

H. J. GELMERS[1], J. H. A. WIEZER[1], C. J. DE WEERDT[1], and K. GORTER[1]

Abstract

Current research suggests that cerebral ischemia induces a cascade of pathophysiological reactions, with a massive influx of calcium into the neuron as the "final common pathway", resulting in catabolism and cell necrosis due to calcium overload. Treatment with calcium entry blockers, therefore, may be a new approach to arresting, and possibly preventing, destruction of cerebral tissue in stroke patients. The calcium entry blocker nimodipine was found to inhibit selectively spasms of the isolated cerebral arteries, produced either by depolarization or by receptor stimulation. In vivo experiments demonstrated that postischemic impairment of cerebral blood flow, which may be a major contributor to neuronal damage, is prevented.

After encouraging, although not conclusive, results of a single-blind pilot study, further clinical studies were undertaken and a double-blind, placebo-controlled, multicenter study was conducted. The data from this study strongly suggest that patients with acute ischemic stroke benefit from treatment with 120 mg nimodipine, started with 24 h after onset, combined with a "standard" treatment, e. g., hemodilution by low molecular weight dextran. The conclusion so far is that calcium entry blockers such as nimodipine, may be useful in the treatment of patients with acute ischemic stroke.

Introduction

This presentation reviews pathophysiological mechanisms in ischemic brain damage, with special reference to recently discussed cascades of metabolic abnormalities, including calcium overload, which can lead to subsequent cell death. The theoretical and experimental background for the application of nimodipine, a calcium antagonist, in brain ischemia and acute stroke is discussed. Reference is made to the authors' experiences with nimodipine treatment in acute stroke patients.

[1] Department of Neurology, Streekziekenhuis, 7607 PP Almelo, The Netherlands

Theories and Facts

Stating the Clinical Problem of Acute Ischemic Stroke

Ischemic stroke may be defined as a focal neurological deficit of abrupt onset, reaching a peak of severity in minutes or hours, usually followed by partial recovery. With respect to the clinical course, ischemic stroke can be divided into four categories: transient ischemic attack, progressing stroke in which the neurological deficit continuously worsens, evolving stroke in which the neurological symptoms are clearing up, and completed stroke in which there is neither improvement nor worsening of the neurological signs during the initial days.

Although great progress has been made in the last few decades in understanding the nature of stroke and the accompanying alterations in cerebral circulation, there is still no definitive therapy available for the patient who has suffered a brain infarction. The main goal in the management of stroke is preventing of the occurrence of a completed stroke by treatment of the progressing stroke or transient ischemic attack. The objective of medical treatment of ischemic stroke is to restore the perfusion of the compromised areas of the brain and to prevent secondary subsequent ischemic events, the latter being destructive reactions involving lipolysis, proteolysis, and failure of intracellular transport (see above). Despite a wealth of experimental data, only limited and often anecdotal information seems to be available on the efficacy of the plethora of therapeutic interventions advocated. Clinicians have believed for many years that the persistence of signs and symptoms of cerebral ischemia for more than a few minutes signified irreversible cellular damage in the brain. This rather pessimistic view, leading to therapeutic nihilism, was challenged by the demonstration that cerebral tissue of several mammalian species was able to survive, at least partially, profound cerebral ischemia lasting 1 h [1].

Mechanism of Ischemic Cell Damage

The realization that the brain is far more resistant to ischemia than previously thought has raised the possibility of intervening in a meaningful way before damage becomes irreversible. Consequently, attention has been focused on a variety of factors that might be of importance in determining irreversible cell damage.

Experiments on focal cerebral ischemia have shown that a progressive reduction of cerebral blood flow (CBF) is associated with increasing glycolysis and a rise in cellular lactate production, while the levels of the high-energy phosphates remain unaltered. Electrical activity progressively diminishes, and the electroencephalographic EEG power and evoked potentials become isoelectric if the flow decreases to less than about 20 ml 100 g^{-1} min^{-1} [2]. This flow level is commonly called the electrical or functional ischemic threshold [3] and is associated with a critical decrease of substrate delivery and a mild rise in extracellular fluid potassium which, paradoxically, stimulates metabolism. In addition, cessation of regular synthesis of neurotransmitters, release of potent vasoconstricting substances, and intravascular coagulation (e. g., eicosanoids) contribute to this

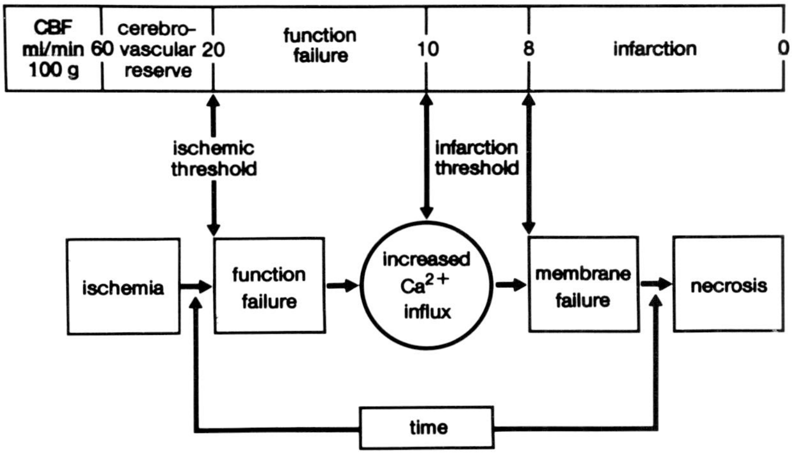

Fig. 1. The ischemic cascade. Values are approximations obtained from experimental data. *CBF*, cerebral blood flow

dangerous state of ischemia. At this stage, however, electrical quiescence is not necessarily synonymous with loss of cell viability.

As soon as the CBF reaches the so-called infarction threshold of about $10-12\ \mathrm{ml}\ 100\ \mathrm{g}^{-1}\ \mathrm{min}^{-1}$, membrane depolarization due to extensive potassium efflux occurs. At the same time, calcium influx into the cells begins (Fig. 1), thus activating different self-propagating energy-wasting cycles. Once the regulatory system breaks down, high-energy phosphate levels fall rapidly. Calcium influx also unleashes destructive reactions involving lipolysis (with production of free fatty acids including arachidonic acid) and proteolysis, resulting in receptor dysfunction and failure of intracellular transport mechanisms. Influx of calcium into mitochondria leads to the breakdown of their function. Damage to the organelles is one further step towards irreversible neuronal death [4, 5].

Brain tissue next to an infarcted area is underperfused and physiologically very labile. This area is named the penumbra [3]. Its perfusion pattern may be patchy with multiple small infarcted areas surrounded by surviving but quiescent cells. Therapy is aimed at rescuing "nonfunctional" but not definitely infarcted tissue, in order to reduce the area of infarction as well as to minimize the neurological deficits.

Role of Calcium Entry Blockers in Brain Ischemia

An exciting advance in the treatment of brain ischemia has been initiated by the introduction of drugs that, at least in vitro, block calcium entry into cells. Calcium entry blockers comprise a rather heterogeneous group of drugs, and include derivatives of papavarine, dihydropyridine, and piperazine. Currently, there is not yet sufficient information on the whole pharmacological profile of most calcium entry blockers. Some have additional effects not related to the influences on calcium. This also explains the difficulties in classification [6].

Nimodipine is a dihydropyridine derivative with specific effects on the cerebrovascular system. In isolated vessels, nimodipine inhibits spasms induced by depolarization independently of the original site of the vascular bed [7] and, in addition, selectively inhibits spasms induced by spasmogenic agonists like serotonin, catecholamines, histamine, thromboxanes, or whole blood [8] in isolated cerebral vessels.

Experimental Studies with Nimodipine

The relevance of these in vitro findings has been investigated in experimental models of brain ischemia. The effect of nimodipine on cerebrovascular reactivity was shown in studies with so-called stroke-prone rats [9]. Long-term treatment with nimodipine largely prevented the occurrence of strokes and damage to vessels and brain parenchyma, as well as the associated deaths of stroke-prone rats. It could be demonstrated that this was not due to the effect of reduction of blood pressure. The effects of nimodipine bolus injections of $1-100\ \mu g\ kg^{-1}$ (i. v.) on the cardiovascular system of dogs were studied [14]. Blood pressure decreased, cardiac output and coronary sinus oxygen saturation increased. There was either no or only a slight reduction of the heart rate, probably due to an effect on baroreceptor reflexes.

In cats, nimodipine prevented postischemic secondary underperfusion after transient interruption of the cerebral circulation [10, 11], while in dogs there was a remarkable improvement of neurological deficits caused by total cerebral ischemia induced by ligation of the aorta [12]. Similar studies were performed in primates (pigtailed monkeys [13]). They were subjected to a 17-min period of complete cerebral ischemia and then treated with nimodipine 10 μg/kg (as an intravenous bolus) over 2 min followed by an infusion of $1\ \mu g\ kg^{-1}\ min^{-1}$ for 10 h. The neurological outcome 96 h after ischemia was significantly better in nimodipine-treated animals than in untreated animals.

Clinical Studies with Nimodipine

Effect on Cerebral Blood Flow. In acute stroke, the hemisphere involved has decreased perfusion, as can be demonstrated by reliable techniques for measuring CBF. Within the ischemic hemisphere, the perfusion rate may vary from region to region, and focal areas of decreased CBF tend to occur within the infarcted area, whereas hyperemic regions may sometimes be found at the periphery of the infarction [15]. The presence of hyperemic areas is called the "luxury perfusion syndrome" and has been attributed to local metabolism [16].

Autoregulation, defined as the inherent ability of the cerebral vasculature to maintain a constant blood flow through a wide range of cerebral perfusion pressures, is often lost after a stroke, and CBF becomes totally pressure dependent. Normal autoregulatory function may return within days or weeks after the ischemic episode. In addition, the normal response to cerebral tissue carbon dioxide partial pressure may be decreased or absent, and paradoxical reactions may occur. The latter is known as the "intracerebral steal phenomenon" and is characterized by a further decrease in CBF in the ischemic region in response to carbon dioxide or any other vasodilatory trigger [17, 18].

CBF measurements in healthy volunteers revealed a small dose-dependent increase in mean hemispheric blood flow after nimodipine [19]. In patients with acute ischemic stroke, the effect on mean hemispheric blood flow was less pronounced and was not or only just significant [19, 20]. In the affected and underperfused regions, a favorable effect was indicated by a significant increase of regional CBF. This increase in underperfused affected regions, without any distinct effect on the circulation elsewhere in the brain, at least suggests that no steal effect will occur with nimodipine.

Effect in Acute Stroke. In a single-blind pilot study of 60 acute stroke patients, 31 were treated with a "standard" therapy (see below) and 29 with nimodipine (120 mg daily for a period of 4 weeks) in addition to the standard therapy [21]. The neurological deficit of patients receiving nimodipine improved faster and showed a statistically significant improvement in comparison with standard therapy patients after a 4-week study period. Heart rate decreased with nimodipine therapy and increased on standard treatment alone, whereas only a very mild difference in blood pressure was noted between the two treatment regimens.

These results were sufficiently encouraging to prompt a double-blind, placebo-controlled, multicenter study [22]. All patients were admitted to hospital within 24 h (most of them even within 8 h), and (for ethical reasons) all received a "standard" treatment comprising 500 ml low molecular weight dextran (i. v.) administered over 12 h each day for 5 days and intensive supportive care involving intensive nursing, physiotherapy, logopedics, and occupational therapy. In addition, after randomization, the patients received either 120 mg nimodipine or placebo for 28 days. Cardiotonic, antihypertensive medications, and antibiotics were administered if required, whereas steroids, vasodilators, or anticoagulants were avoided. Neurological deficits were assessed using the Mathew scale for neurological scoring. Of the 186 patients included, 164 were valid for evaluation of efficacy (the main reason for exclusion was lack of confirmation of ischemic stroke by cranial computed tomography). Of these, 79 received nimodipine and 85 placebo. The mean age and age distribution of both groups were very similar, as was the distribution of risk factors.

Table 1. Mathew sum score after 4 weeks in patients with initial scores of 35 – 65 (severe deficit, 59% of all patients)

	Placebo ($n = 46$)	Nimodipine ($n = 49$)
Sum score >91	10.9%	12.2%
Sum score 66 – 90	37.0%	51.0%
Sum score 35 – 65	23.9%	28.6%
Sum score <35	2.2%	–
Died	26.1%	8.2%

$p = 0.003$ (Mantel-Cox). From [20]

Table 2. Performance or disability status after 4 weeks in patients with initial scores of 7 (severe sequelae, 65% of all patients)

Disability score (0 – 28)		Placebo ($n = 52$)	Nimodipine ($n = 53$)
Normal	(= 28)	5.8%	9.4%
Mild	(= 21)	11.5%	30.2%
Moderate	(= 14)	30.8%	28.3%
Severe	(= 7)	23.1%	22.6%
Died	(= 0)	28.8%	9.4%

$p = 0.046$ (Mantel-Cox). From [20]

One of the major parameters of the study was the mortality rate after 4 weeks. In the nimodipine group, six patients died, compared with 18 of the 85 placebo patients. This would imply a significant advantage of treatment with nimodipine. Even more important was the improvement of the neurological deficits with nimodipine (see Tables 1, 2).

Nimodipine was generally well tolerated at the doses used in this study, and there were no major effects on blood pressure or the mean heart rate. Adverse side effects were minimal, except for one patient who developed moderate renal insufficiency. It remains doubtful, however, whether this was a result of nimodipine or of low molecular weight dextran.

Conclusion

Recently, the important role of calcium in the pathophysiology of ischemic cell damage has been the focus of considerable investigation and discussion. During ischemia, a cascade of pathophysiological reactions occur, finally resulting in a massive influx of calcium in neurons [23]. Ultimately, this leads to a calcium overload with subsequent neuronal death. Treatment with calcium entry blockers therefore seems to offer a new approach to arresting, and possibly preventing, destruction of cerebral tissue in stroke patients. Experimental data support this view. After a pilot study with promising results, a full clinical trial was conducted. Much thought was given to the methodology of this study because no satisfactory stroke trial has as yet been undertaken [24]. A double-blind, randomized, placebo-controlled, multicenter design was chosen. It is perhaps unrealistic to expect administration of a single agent to influence outcome significantly after severe brain ischemia, and it is almost certain that multiple therapeutic interventions will be required [25]. For this reason, as well as for ethical reasons, it was decided, despite methodological objections, to administer the drug on trial in addition to a "standard" treatment. Among the difficulties to be resolved in designing a stroke trial are selection and definition of the assessment criteria. Views of how to measure the efficacy of a drug in a stroke trial differ. The Mathew scale has proved a good tool for assessing neurological deficits in patients with acute stroke and correlates well with patients' conditions [26, 27]. The interobserver agreement between the neurologists at the participating centers was estimated in a separate study (H. J. Gelmers, K. Gorter, C. J. de Weerdt, and H. J. A. Wiezer, unpublished data) and found to be good enough to avoid confounding of data analysis.

From this multicenter stroke trial, we can draw no definite conclusions regarding the pharmacological mechanism by which the improvement was achieved, since two therapies were used simultaneously. It is tempting to speculate that nimodipine, as a calcium entry blocker with selective action on cerebral vessels, may serve as a protective agent in cerebral ischemia, aborting or retarding the metabolic consequences of the ischemic insult, while low molecular weight dextran, a well-documented therapy to improve postischemic hypoperfusion, influences hemorrheological factors [28].

The conclusion so far is that additional treatment of patients with acute ischemic stroke with the new calcium entry blocker nimodipine benefits these patients with respect to mortality and severity of neurological deficits and has few if any unwanted side effects.

References

1. Hossmann KA, Zimmerman V (1974) Resuscitation of brain after one hour of complete ischemia. Brain Res 81:59–74
2. Astrup J, Symon L, Branston NM, Lassen NA (1979) Cortical evoked potentials of brain ischemia. Stroke 8:51–57
3. Astrup J, Siesjo BK, Symon L (1981) Thresholds in cerebral ischemia. The ischemic penumbra. Stroke 12:723–725
4. Siesjo BK (1981) Cell damage in the brain: a speculative hypothesis. J Cereb Blood Flow Metab 1:155–186
5. Hass WK (1981) Beyond cerebral blood flow, metabolism and ischemic thresholds: an examination of the role of calcium in the initiation of cerebral infarction. In: Meyer JS, Lechner H, Reivich M, Ott EO, Arabinar A (eds) Cerebral vascular disease, vol 3, Proceedings of the 10th Salzburg conference on cerebral vascular disease. Exerpta Medica, Amsterdam, pp 3–17
6. Godfraind T (1984) Basic mechanisms and classification of calcium entry blockers. In: Godfraind T, Herman AG, Wellens D (eds) Calcium entry blockers in cardiovascular and cerebral dysfunctions. Martinus Nijhoff, The Hague, pp 9–18
7. Towart R (1981) The selective inhibition of serotonin-induced contractions of rabbit cerebral vascular smooth muscle by calcium-antagonistic dihydropyridines. Circ Res 18:650–657
8. White RP, Cunningham MP, Robertson JT (1982) Effect of the calcium antagonist nimodipine on the contractile responses of isolated canine basilar arteries induced by serotonin, prostaglandin F2a, thrombin and whole blood. Neurosurgery 10:344–348
9. Kazda S, Garthoff B, Luckhaus G (1983) Calcium antagonists prevent brain damage in stroke prone spontaneously hypertensive rats. J Cereb Blood Flow Metab 3:526–527
10. Kazda S, Hoffmeister F (1979) Effect of some cerebral vasodilators on the postischemic impaired cerebral perfusion in cats. Acta Pharmacol (Suppl)307:R43
11. Kazda S, Garthoff B, Krause WP, Schlossman K (1982) Cerebrovascular effects of the calcium antagonistic dihydropyridine derivate nimodipine in animal experiments. Arzneimittelforsch 32:331–338
12. Steen PA, Newberg LA, Milde JH, Michenfelder JD (1983) Nimodipine improves cerebral blood flow and neurologic recovery after complete ischemia in the dog. J Cereb Blood Flow Metab 3:38–43
13. Newberg LA, Steen PA, Milde JH et al. (1984) Effects of nimodipine on cerebral blood flow and neurologic function following complete global ischemia in dogs and primates. In: Betz E, Deck K, Hoffmeister F (eds) First international nimotop symposium. Schattauer, Stuttgart, pp 99–104

14. Taylor DG, Kowalski TE (1984) Comparison of calcium channel inhibitors on vagal heart rate responses elicited by arterial baroreceptor reflexes in anaesthesized dogs. J Pharmacol Exp Ther 228:491–499
15. Paulson OB, Lassen NA, Skinhøj E (1970) Regional cerebral blood flow in apoplexy without arterial occlusion. Neurology 20:125–138
16. Lassen NA (1966) The luxury perfusion syndrome and its possible relation to acute metabolic acidosis localised within the brain. Lancet ii:1113–1116
17. Fieschi C, Aguoli A, Principe M, Battistini N, Bozzao L, Nardini M (1969) Impairment of the regional vasomotor response of central vessels to hypercarbia in vascular diseases. Eur Neurol 2:13–20
18. Paulson OB, Lassen MA, Skinhøj E (1970) Regional cerebral blood flow in apoplexy without atrial occlusion. Neurology 20:125–138
19. Gaab MR, Brawanski A, Bockhorn J, Maximilian VA (1982) Calcium antagonism: a new therapeutic principle in stroke and cerebral vasospasm? Reg Cerebral Blood Flow Bull (Novo Copenhagen) 3:47–51
20. Gelmers HJ (1982) Effect of nimodipine on postischemic cerebrovascular reactivity, as revealed by measuring regional cerebral blood flow (rCBF). Acta Neurochir 63:283–290
21. Gelmers HJ (1984) The effect of nimodipine on the clinical course of patients with acute ischemic stroke. Acta Neurol Scand 69:232–239
22. Gelmers HJ, Gorter K, de Weerdt CJ, Wiezer HJA (1985) Acute ischemic stroke: a controlled trial with the calcium antagonist nimodipine. J Cereb Blood Flow Metab 5(suppl 1):S337
23. Schanne FAK, Kane AB, Young EE et al. (1979) Calcium dependence of toxic cell death: a final common path. Science 20:700–702
24. Capildeo R, Haberman S, Rose CF (1982) Stroke trials: the facts. In: Rose CF (ed) Advances in stroke therapy. Raven, New York, pp 53–62
25. Hinds CJ (1985) Brain ischemia. Br Med J 291:758–760
26. Mathew NT, Meyer JS, Rivera VH (1972) Double blind evaluation of glycerol treatment in acute cerebral infarction. Lancet ii:1327–1333
27. Gelmers HJ (1975) Effect of glycerol treatment on the natural history of acute cerebral infarction. Clin Neurol Neurosurg 78:277–282
28. Wood JH, Kee DB Jr (1985) Hemorrheology of the cerebral circulation in stroke. Stroke 16:765–772

Closing Remarks

J. MARSHALL

As you can imagine, I attend many cerebrovascular mettings, but I think it has been some time since I have attended one which has been as stimulating as this. What I have found most stimulating has been the analytical and critical approach which has characterized the contributions here.

Cerebrovascular disease had been much neglected before becoming in the 1950s, for various reasons, an "in" subject. People then began to work on it, and, of course, the answers initially came fairly easily. But then, as with all scientific subjects, the going got tough as time went by, and in the face of this researchers seem to me currently in something of a retreat.

There was a recent article in the *Lancet* suggesting that we conduct a national trial in England specifically on stroke. Patients would have a scan, certainly, to exclude hemorrhages, but the rest of the patients would be considered simply as "strokes" quite irrespective of the cause. Patients would be divided into four groups, those receiving aspirin, beta blockers, aspirin plus beta blockers or placebo. This proposal depressed me very much because it seems to me a reversion to the old days and to treating a phenomenon rather than trying to treat a pathogenetic entity. The argument was that those in public health would be very interested in discovering whether the health of the nation would be better if we relied on aspirin. However, we are not public health people; we are, first of all, clinical physicians, concerned with the best treatment for individual patients. Our first question must therefore be, "What will we do for this patient?" And secondly, as scientific physicians we try to understand what is going on behind the phenomena that we observe.

I think that we have done both during this meeting and in this book. In the *diagnostic* papers, we have heard of numerous sonographic and scintigraphic methods for getting more precisely at the pathogenetic mechanism of stroke. For instance, the contribution on scanning was not concerned merely with the images themselves, but also with what the images tell us about the underlying pathogenesis. The paper on thrombosis did not merely talk about thrombosis as a whole but detailed various subcategories regarding points which we ought to take notice of. This approach was continued in the subsequent contributions with a critical attitude to therapy. We very often use particular therapies because we must do something for the patient. Nevertheless, we are well aware of the lack of our knowledge and the shortcomings concerning these therapeutic procedures.

---

[1] Institute of Neurology, National Hospital for Nervous Diseases, Queen Square, London WC1N 3BG, UK

I think this book, therefore, is a stimulating contribution to the literature on strokes, largely because of its critical and analytical approach to the subject and because it avoids the current trend toward conducting ever bigger and better multicenter trials. This is not to suggest that there is anything wrong with a multicenter trial as such, but multicenter trials tend to regard only phenomena rather than searching for pathogenetic mechanisms.

We would thank Professor Poeck, Professor Ringelstein, and Professor Hacke for organizing such an excellent symposium and for editing these proceedings. We are also grateful for the administrative arrangements which are always very necessary and which have been very successful. We are also indebted to the interpreters and projectionists for their efficient work and, of course, to Bayer for their sponsorship in making it possible. I hope we will take from these papers an improved understanding as a basis for precise diagnoses, and for providing the best treatment we can devise.

Subject Index